getting into the
PHYSICIAN
ASSISTANT
school
of your choice

SECOND EDITION

Andrew J. Rodican, PA-C

McGraw-Hill

Medical Publishing Division

New York Chicago San Francisco Lisbon London Madrid Mexico City Milan
New Delhi San Juan Seoul Singapore Sydney Toronto

Getting Into the Physician Assistant School of Your Choice, Second Edition

1 2 3 4 5 6 7 8 9 0   CUS/CUS   0 9 8 7 6 5 4 3

ISBN 0-07-142185-8

Notice

Medicine is an ever-changing science. As new research and clinical experience broaden our knowledge, changes in treatment and drug therapy are required. The author and the publisher of this work have checked with sources believed to be reliable in their efforts to provide information that is complete and generally in accord with the standards accepted at the time of publication. However, in view of the possibility of human error or changes in medical sciences, neither the author nor the publisher nor any other party who has been involved in the preparation or publication of this work warrants that the information contained herein is in every respect accurate or complete, and they disclaim all responsibility for any errors or omissions or for the results obtained from use of the information contained in this work. Readers are encouraged to confirm the information contained herein with other sources. For example and in particular, readers are advised to check the product information sheet included in the package of each drug they plan to administer to be certain that the information contained in this work is accurate and that changes have not been made in the recommended dose or in the contraindications for administration. This recommendation is of particular importance in connection with new or infrequently used drugs.

This book was set in Goudy by Westchester Book Composition.
The editor was Michael Brown.
The production supervisor was Catherine Saggese.
Project management was provided by Westchester Book Services.
Von Hoffman Graphics was the printer and binder.

This book is printed on acid-free paper.

Library of Congress Cataloging-in-Publication Data

Rodican, Andrew J.
    Getting into the physician assistant school of your choice / Andrew J. Rodican—2nd ed.
        p.   cm.
    Previously published by Appleton & Lange in 1998 as: Getting into the PA school of your choice.
        ISBN 0-07-142185-8 (softcover)
1. Physicians' assistants—Education—United States. 2. Physicians' assistants—Vocational guidance. 3. Medical colleges—United States—Admission.   I. Rodican, Andrew J. Getting into the PA school of your choice.   II. Title.
    R697.P45R646   2003
610.69'53'071173—dc21

                                                                                        2003046455

Please tell the author and publisher of this book by sending your comments to *pa@mcgraw-hill.com*. Please put the author and title of the book in the subject line.

This book is dedicated to the memory of my father,
James A. Rodican

Acknowledgments

This book is a work of passion and was conceived from a simple idea given to me in 1995 by my good friend Charles E. ("Chuck") Ruotolo. For his continued friendship and support I am extremely grateful.

Mom, Aurora ("Nikki") Kreilheim, you are a pillar of strength and my inspiration for becoming a PA. I admire your courage to persevere in the face of adversity. Your best advice to me as a mother, and a nurse, was, "Never forget that good medicine doesn't just come in little bottles and boxes, but in the heart and feelings of the caregiver." Thanks mom, I love you.

Edward ("Eddie") Rodican, my son. I am awed by your intelligence, your cooperative style, and the way you have always stood by me. I cannot express in words how proud I am that you are my son. Your courage to follow your childhood dream is a power of example to me and many others. Aim high, and never give up.

Nicole ("Nikki") Rodican, my daughter. You are a daddy's girl all the way; thank God! Your strength and focus overwhelm me. You have a heart of gold and a singing voice that brings tears of pride to my eyes. You give me strength. Never change.

John Willard, my lifelong friend. We've been through the mill together. Thanks to you (and Lori) for being my friend and for always being there when I needed you most.

Pol ("Flip") Plancon, my mentor and friend. When I met you, the possibility of writing another book was unthinkable. Your support, guidance, and friendship over the past couple of years, along with the support of your wife, Gale, helped me walk through my fears and live life *happily, joyously, and freely*. Thank you for saving my life.

My "crew," Rikki, Eddie, Jimmy, and Liz. Thanks for all of your help and support over the past few years.

Paula Forlano, thank you for helping me with last-minute editing of the second edition, and especially for your friendship.

Pam Filip, thanks for believing in me when I could not believe in myself.

About the Author

Andrew J. Rodican, PA-C, is a former member of the Yale University School of Medicine, Physician Associate Program Admission's Committee. He has interviewed many PA school applicants, and read and evaluated numerous applications. He is a recipient of the Yale University School of Medicine Physician Associate Program 1994 Medical Writing Award, and he is the writer and developer of the seminar, "Getting Into the PA School of Your Choice." He has an extensive sales background, and won the Dale Carnegie Sales Training Course, Sales Talk Championship and Human Relations Award. He combines his broad knowledge of the admissions process with his sales background to maximize each candidate's potential for acceptance into the PA school of his/her choice.

Contents

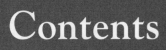

Foreword

A friend and colleague recently asked me to write the foreword to the second edition of his book, *Getting into the Physician Assistant School of Your Choice*. I have known the author, Andrew J. (Andy) Rodican, for the past seven years as a PA student preceptor, co-worker, colleague, and friend. We work together at Concentra Health Services, the largest national provider of occupational medicine to corporations and workers in the United States.

Andy brings to his readers a number of life experiences in the following settings: clinical medicine, business, education, and the health care field. He has a background in medical writing, such as: *Getting into the PA School of Your Choice* (Appleton & Lange/McGraw-Hill), *More Questions than Answers: Hepatitis C Virus in the Nineties* (Presented at Yale University School of Medicine in 1994), and *The Injury Report*, a medical-legal newsletter he developed for workers' compensation and personal injury attorneys in the state of Connecticut. Andy's medical experiences range from that of a former Navy Corpsman to being a PA in cardiovascular surgery. He is the owner of Sound Medical-Legal Consulting, LLC, a consulting firm in Connecticut. Andy Rodican is also a well-known lecturer and has presented his seminar, *Getting into the PA School of Your Choice*, throughout the country. He has acted as a PA preceptor in conjunction with the Yale University School of Medicine and Quinnipiac University PA programs. While working at the Hospital of Saint Raphael in New Haven, Connecticut, he functioned as a Patient Relations Representative for two years. Andy likes to think "outside the box" and he has an entrepreneurial view of the health care field.

Let me categorically state that no book will ever, ever guarantee your success in any endeavor. Books, at best, will provide you with a game plan. It is the game plan, your grades, your qualifications, and your hard work that will lead you on the road to success. In my opinion, *Getting into the Physician Assistant School of Your Choice* will put you on the right road. After reading Andy's book, you will be in a much better position when applying to PA programs. The book tells you, as an applicant, how to work a well-designed game plan, crossing all of the Ts and dotting all of the Is.

Today there are approximately 136 accredited PA programs, with 40% of these programs at the master's level. Whatever level PA program you choose to apply to, the information in this book will assist you on your road to success. I have seen the PA profession grow from a certificate-type program to a master's level profession. Over the past 35-plus years in which the profession has been in existence, we have made tremendous strides and exceeded even our own expectations. I expect that we will continue to make greater strides over the next 35 years.

I encourage and commend you on your efforts to enter the PA profession and this book will help you do so. Your quest begins with your picking up this book and seeing what the author has to offer you. Remember the old Chinese saying: *A journey of 10,000 miles begins with the first step*. This book is your first step!

I wish you luck on your journey, and on your road to success in applying to PA schools.

George F. (Rick) Hillegas, PA-C, MPH
Assistant Professor
Quinnipiac University

George F. (Rick) Hillegas, PA-C, MPH, has a varied life experience. He completed a career in the military and has been a medical practitioner, a college professor, and, most recently, a candidate for public office in the state of Connecticut. Life and challenges along with strong religious and ethical beliefs have been a part of his personality and character.

Rick spent twenty-six years in military service. He initially served as an enlisted hospital corpsman in the Navy, where he trained as a surgical technician and field medic for the Marines. This proved to be a life-changing experience and further directed him into the caring professions. He often says that the military was one of the greatest educational experiences he has had in his life. In fact, it was because of his military medical experience that he chose to become a physician assistant. Prior to leaving the military, he was accepted into three foreign medical schools. In the final analysis, he was accepted to, and chose to attend, the first class of PA students at the George Washington University Medical School in 1972.

From 1975–1992 Rick served as a warrant officer in the Coast Guard. While on active duty he completed his master's in public health at the University of California at Berkeley. Rick was awarded a yearlong Congressional Health Policy Fellowship, sponsored by Burrows-Welcome pharmaceuticals and the American Academy of Physician Assistants (AAPA). He served in the office of Congressman Jim McDermott as a health policy fellow and as a congressional aide. Upon completing the fellowship, he entered academia and became very active in PA politics early on in this career forum.

In 1994, Rick took a position at the Quinnipiac University PA program as an assistant professor and clinical coordinator. For the past six years, Rick has held the position of vice-president for the Quinnipiac Faculty Federation and has been a member of the Faculty Senate for four years.

During the 2000 election cycle, Rick threw his hat into the ring and ran for the Connecticut State Senate. His first time out of the box, Rick had an impressive showing, garnering 40% of the vote. He is being encouraged to run again by the Republican Party of the State of Connecticut. Rick feels, "In one form or another we are all politicians and salesmen."

Preface

There is no security on this earth. There is only opportunity.

—General Douglas MacArthur

This is the second edition of *Getting into the PA School of Your Choice*. The first edition was published in 1997, and at that time there were approximately 2,500 (graduating) physician assistant (PA) students enrolled in 98 PA programs throughout the United States. At the time of this writing, there are approximately 4,200 (graduating) PA students enrolled in 136 programs in the country.

In 1996, there were 30,000 practicing physician assistants and the U.S. Department of Labor projected a 36% increase in the number of PA jobs by the year 2005. By 2001, however, the number of PAs in practice already reached 45,000, representing a 50% increase in jobs in just less than five years.

The future continues to look bright for PAs. The profession currently ranks twelfth on the Bureau of Labor Statistics' (BLS) list of fastest-growing occupations from 2000–2010, and it projects that PA jobs will increase by 53% by the year 2010.

Because this book has become the definitive guide for physician assistant applicants and has helped large numbers of people achieve success, many of the basic concepts remain unchanged. The chapter titled *The Essay* and most of the *Interview* chapters are left intact, since they encompass the backbone of the admissions process.

In response to feedback from applicants who read the first volume and to comments from those who attended the author's national seminars, the second edition contains three new chapters: *What Do PA Programs Look for in an Applicant?*, *The Internet for PA School Applicants*, and a revised *The Interview (Part One)* chapter containing the interview experience of a PA friend and colleague.

All changes in the second edition are consistent with the mission of the first edition: to help the best-qualified applicants achieve success by gaining a full understanding of the admissions process. If you have a strong desire to become a physician assistant, I hope that you will find in this book a comprehensive plan for reaching your dream.

List of Contributors

Karin Augur, PA-C

Linda Hricz-Borges, PA-C

George Brothers, PA-C

J.M. Farrell, PA-C

Rick Hillegas, PA-C

Rosemary Jones

Don Solomini, PA-C

Terry Spahr, PA-C

Introduction
So You Want to Be a Physician Assistant

Perhaps you always wanted to practice medicine, but did not want to invest the time and money necessary to become a physician.

You want a medical career that will challenge you intellectually, reward you emotionally and financially, yet still enable you to spend quality time with your family or pursue outside interests. Whether you always wanted to be a PA or you are just testing the waters, you have taken the first step.

Many of us once dreamed of becoming physicians. Then, for various reasons, our priorities and circumstances changed. Some of us cannot afford to put life on hold for the eight or more years it takes to become a physician. Our family dynamics during undergraduate school—divorce, death, etc.— may have had a negative impact on our GPA, making us less than ideal candidates for medical school. Maybe you came to realize that as a PA you will have more time to practice medicine and not have to be concerned with the business aspect of running a medical practice.

Some of us gravitate toward medicine years after completing our undergraduate work. Maybe we did some volunteer work in a hospital, or perhaps know a PA who may have inspired us. Some of us are drawn to the PA profession after a life-changing event. Whatever your motivation is for applying to PA school, this book will place you well on the path to reaching your goal.

HOW DID THE PA PROFESSION BEGIN?

Dr. Eugene Stead of the Duke University Medical Center in North Carolina is considered the pioneer of the PA profession and started the first PA program in 1965. The profession got its start because of a shortage and disproportionate distribution of primary care physicians at the time. The first program was comprised of former Navy corpsmen who served in Vietnam and already had considerable clinical experience. These former corpsmen had no venue for transferring their skills to the civilian world. Dr. Stead trained these corpsmen, comparable to the fast-track programs physicians completed during World War II. The profession grew from these first few veterans to over 45,000 practicing PAs today.

WHAT IS A PHYSICIAN ASSISTANT?

Physician assistants are health care professionals licensed to practice medicine with physician supervision. Rather than follow their physician colleagues around by the proverbial coattails, however, most PAs work autonomously and, typically, collaboratively with their MD supervisors. PAs are broadly trained and perform a variety of duties depending on the specialty, practice setting, supervising physician, and scope of practice. In general, PAs perform a comprehensive history and physical examination, formulate a diagnosis and treatment plan, order and interpret diagnostic tests, assist in surgery, prescribe medications, counsel patients and family, perform minor surgical procedures, and consult with their supervising physicians.

PAs are found in almost every area and specialty of medical and surgical practice. About half of all PAs work in primary care (family practice, obstetrics and gynocology, pediatrics, and internal medicine). Another 20% work in the various surgical specialties, and the remainder of PAs work in a host of other specialty and subspecialty arenas. Some PAs actually own their own practice and hire a supervising physician to work for them.

The mean PA is 42 years old, and the profession is almost equally divided between men and women. A new graduate can expect to earn approximately $60,000 per year to start. The average PA probably earns about $72,000 to $75,000 per year. Many PAs, depending on experience and scope of practice, earn over $100,000 per year. Slightly over two-thirds of all PAs have a bachelor's degree, and slightly less than one-third of all PAs have a master's degree. Few PAs have a doctorate degree.

> **PAs ARE FOUND IN ALMOST EVERY AREA AND SPECIALTY OF MEDICAL AND SURGICAL PRACTICE.**
>
> **THE MEAN PA IS 42 YEARS OLD, AND THE PROFESSION IS ALMOST EQUALLY DIVIDED BETWEEN MEN AND WOMEN.**

HOW ARE PAs TRAINED?

Most PA programs are approximately two years in length. Students are trained in the *medical model,* similar to most medical school programs. In fact, the didactic phase of a PA program is often equated to the first three years of medical school. Many PA students share certain classes with medical students at those programs affiliated with a medical school. The main difference between physician training and physician assistant training is the number of years physicians are required to spend in a residency after the didactic phase is completed.

The first year of PA school is typically dedicated to the classroom and clinical practicum sessions. PA students can expect to take courses in clinical laboratory services, electrocardiography, emergency medicine and trauma, interviewing techniques, medicine and surgery, microbiology and infectious disease, pharmacology, physical examination, physiology and biochemistry, psychodynamics of human behavior, anatomy, diagnostic imaging, epidemiology and public health, ethics, human sexuality, and pathology.

The second year is geared toward clinical rotations. Most programs have mandatory rotations in emergency medicine, family/general medicine, general surgery, internal medicine, obstetrics and gynecology, pediatrics, and psychiatry. In addition, students can typically choose from a number of elective rotations.

Upon graduating from an accredited PA program, the student is eligible to sit for the national certifying examination, which is given by the National Commission on Certification of Physician Assistants (NCCPA) in conjunction with the National Board of Medical Examiners. The student is eligible for state licensure after passing the national examination. PAs must acquire 100 hours of continuing medical education (CME) every two years, and pass a national recertification exam every six years.

WHERE IS THE PA PROFESSION HEADED?

The future of the PA profession looks bright. Since 1989, the number of graduating PA students has steadily increased from approximately 1,000 per year to over 4,000 per year as of 2001. The PA profession currently ranks twelfth on the Bureau of Labor Statistics' list of fastest-growing occupations from 2000–2010.

New limits on medical resident's working hours will also increase the demand for hospital-based PAs. The Accreditation Council for Graduate Medical Education (ACGME) announced new rules to restrict physician resident's work weeks, starting in July, 2003. Medical residents are restricted to working only 80 hours per week. The result of this change should increase the demand for PAs nationwide. A prominent physician at Yale-New Haven Hospital labeled this new edict the *PA Employment Act*.

THE TYPICAL PA SCHOOL APPLICANT

The admissions committee for any given PA program reviews hundreds of applications each year for as few as 30 to 40 available slots. The admissions process is extremely competitive and therefore the applicant should meet minimum criteria. Ideally, the applicant should satisfy all of the prerequisites of a particular program prior to applying. This includes academic and clinical experience. Most applicants have a bachelor's degree and about four to five years of hands-on clinical experience. SAT/GRE scores of those accepted tend to be in the above-average range.

Keep in mind, however, that looking good on paper is only one part of the equation. In the next chapter I am going to introduce you to the five qualities that will make you a strong, competitive PA school applicant.

THE PA PROFESSION CURRENTLY RANKS TWELFTH ON THE BUREAU OF LABOR STATISTICS' LIST OF FASTEST-GROWING OCCUPATIONS FROM 2000–2010.

What Do PA Programs Look for in an Applicant?

Luck is when preparedness meets opportunity.

—*Author unknown*

At the time of this writing there are 136 accredited PA programs in the United States. If you were to interview admissions committee members from each program, you would probably get 136 differing opinions and ideas on what the committee looks for in a PA school applicant. Fortunately, there are some basic criteria that all programs follow to evaluate candidates for admission. The five basic categories include:

► Passion
► Academic ability and test scores
► Medical experience
► Understanding of the PA profession
► Maturity

In this chapter, we will consider each of these five categories.

PASSION

Passion is the fuel that can propel an otherwise average candidate to the top of the applicant pool. Passion is the burning desire of emotion that motivates an applicant to study that extra hour, take that additional chemistry course, or gain that extra year of hands-on medical experience before applying to PA school. Passion takes the words *I can't* right out of your vocabulary and replaces them with *I will*. Passion cannot be taught; it must come from deep wthin.

The applicant who is passionate about becoming a PA will begin to take certain steps on her own. She finds the time to locate and shadow PAs in her community. She reads PA journals and becomes aware of issues and trends in the PA profession. She has a crystal-clear vision of what the PA role is all about and can verbalize exactly why she wants to become a PA rather than a physician or a nurse practitioner.

A key benefit of having passion is the motivation it provides. On Saturday nights, when you would prefer to be out with your friends rather than studying pharmacology or microbiology, your passion for knowledge will keep you focused. On clinical rotations, when you are spending nights in the

PASSION TAKES THE WORDS *I CAN'T* RIGHT OUT OF YOUR VOCABULARY AND REPLACES THEM WITH *I WILL*.

on-call room rather than sleeping in your own bed, your passion for practical experience will make it all seem worthwhile.

The admissions committee can sense your passion from your essay or from simply looking you in the eye at the interview. Think about why you really want to become a PA, and try to incorporate that passion into the entire application process.

ACADEMIC ABILITY AND TESTS SCORES

PA school applicants frequently want to know the magic grade point average (GPA) or SAT score needed to gain acceptance to a PA program. Many applicants falsely assume that they must possess a 4.0 GPA and 1500 SAT scores to be competitive candidates. This simply isn't true. In fact, the average applicant probably falls somewhere between a 3.0 and 3.2 GPA, with SAT scores in the 1000 to 1100 range.

It is important, though, that a candidate demonstrates a reasonable aptitude in the "hard" sciences. Ultimately, the committee will want to be sure that you can manage a didactically challenging program that encompasses graduate level coursework in anatomy and physiology, biochemistry, and the pathophysiology of the disease process. If you had a difficult time with undergraduate chemistry and biology, you will surely struggle in PA school. Competition is intense, and although the committee may overlook a grade of C in U.S. History or Spanish I, they will be less tolerant of a marginal grade in the sciences.

The good news is that the committee considers trends rather than absolute numbers. For instance, the student who has a few Cs, or even a D, as a freshman can make a favorable impression on the committee if he rebounded with As and Bs in his junior and senior years. In fact, the student who continues to improve will fair much better than the student who trends downward.

To further illustrate the point let's look at the undergraduate science grades of two hypothetical applicants, Mary and Bob:

	Mary	**Bob**
Freshman:	General Chemistry: D+	General Chemistry: A
	Microbiology: C	Microbiology: A
Sophomore:	Organic Chemistry: C	Organic Chemistry: A
	Biochemistry: B	Biochemistry: B
Junior:	Inorganic Chemistry: B	Inorganic Chemistry: B
	Cell Biology: A	Cell Biology: C
Senior:	Physical Chemistry: A	Physical Chemistry: D+
	Genetics: A	Genetics: C

Note that both applicants have an identical GPA, approximately 3.0, yet Mary's overall trend is upward, versus Bob's trend, which is downward. Mary would be the stronger candidate with respect to academic performance.

Other factors the committee considers when evaluating a candidate's academic ability include: 1) number of credit hours taken per semester, 2) course difficulty, 3) reputation of the college or university, 4) life's difficulties and circumstances, 5) extracurricular activities. Let's look at each of these factors separately.

Number of credit hours taken per semester. A typical day in PA school may require a student to sit in the classroom for eight to ten hours, attend an early evening physical examination seminar, and study for three to fours more hours that night in preparation for a pharmacology exam the following morning. This daily, rigorous schedule demands excellent time-management skills from the student, as well as an ability to comprehend and assimilate volumes of scientific material. The only means the admissions committee has to evaluate whether you can make the grade in this area is by reviewing your undergraduate transcript. The applicant who carried a full undergraduate course load while working part time will make a more favorable impression on the committee than the applicant who took fewer classes and/or didn't work at all.

Course difficulty. The admissions committee will probably favor the application from a chemistry major who achieved a 3.0 GPA over that of a history major who achieved a higher, 3.3, GPA. This fact should not be surprising to most applicants. It is the committee's job to select those applicants best suited to thrive in a graduate level science program.

Reputation of the college or university. Although this area is highly subjective, the learning institution itself can be a deciding factor in the application process. For example, let's consider two applicants in the running for the last available slot in a class. Mark has a 3.0 GPA in biochemistry from Harvard University. John has an overall 3.7 GPA in biology from a state university, but he also took many of his undergraduate prerequisite science courses at the local community college before transferring to the state university. John's GPA is higher, but Mark will probably get accepted based on the strength and reputation of his undergraduate institution.

Life's difficulties and circumstances. We all experience a variety of trauma in our lives, some of us more than others. The committee will certainly consider unusual circumstances that may have influenced your GPA or other areas of your application. Significant stressors may include divorce, death of a significant other, or a serious medical illness. Although we cannot avoid these special circumstances, and the committee will consider each case individually, it is important to demonstrate how you may have overcome your particular challenge or obstacle and that you are now focused on your goal.

Extracurricular activities. Grades aren't everything. The admissions committee is looking for well-rounded individuals with some quality *life experience*. Be sure to let the committee know if you've been involved with the Peace Corps, if you play in a band, or even if you race motorcycles. Life experience is an invaluable resource to you as a medical professional. We must be able to relate to patients from varied cultures and backgrounds.

Standardized test scores. Suffice it to say that SAT and GRE scores are prerequisites for most programs, but they do not play a significant a role in the admissions process. Standardized test scores only come into play if you've scored exceptionally high or extremely low, and they serve to validate the rest of your application.

MEDICAL EXPERIENCE

PA school applicants come to the table with a variety of medical experience, especially if they're strong applicants. Unfortunately, some applicants have no medical experience at all, which certainly hurts their chances of getting accepted. Most committee members will insist on some prior medical experience before they will consider the applicant as a serious candidate.

GRADES AREN'T EVERYTHING. THE ADMISSIONS COMMITTEE IS LOOKING FOR WELL-ROUNDED INDIVIDUALS WITH SOME QUALITY *LIFE EXPERIENCE.*

On average, four years of prior experience in one of the following areas is common:

Nursing
    Registered Nurse (RN)
    Licensed Practical Nurse (LPN)
    Certified Nursing Assistant (CNA)
Allied Health
    Physical Therapist
    Occupational Therapist
    X-ray Technician
Emergency Services
    Emergency Medical Technician (EMT)
    Paramedic
    Emergency Room Technician
Miscellaneous
    Phlebotomist
    Athletic Trainer
    Medical Researcher
    Medical Volunteer

As mentioned repeatedly in this text, applying to PA school is an extremely competitive process. The more *points* you score with the committee, the better. Think about your own experience and how you might be able to improve upon it. If you have little or no medical experience, consider doing volunteer work at the local hospital or clinic. The more hands-on medical experience you have, the stronger you will be as a candidate.

UNDERSTANDING OF THE PA PROFESSION

The PA profession is one that has enjoyed tremendous growth over the past decade. That trend, according to the U.S. Bureau of Labor Statistics (BLS), is expected to continue for at least another decade. PA salaries are at an all-time high and continue to rise. As a result of these positive factors, applications to the various PA programs remain strong. The challenge facing the admissions committee is to separate the wheat from the chafe, if you will. One way committee members do this is by closely examining each applicant's motivation for becoming a PA and deciding if they have a realistic understanding of the PA profession.

Many applicants view PA school as a stepping-stone to medical school. This is a huge mistake. Although both professions allow the individual to practice medicine, ours is a dependent profession, by definition. We do not want to become MDs. The *MD wannabe* who becomes a PA first will be miserable, and the committee will see right through this tactic.

Be sure you understand what it means to be a dependent practitioner. In other words, unlike nurse practitioners, PAs must always work under the direct supervision of a physician. This does not mean that you will follow your supervising physician around by the coattails, however. In fact, PAs are expected to be fairly autonomous with respect to evaluating and treating their own patients. It is actually a nice benefit, however, to have a supervising physician available for the more difficult, complex cases.

To get a better understanding of the PA profession, try shadowing various PAs who work in different specialties. Most PAs will be excited about your interest in the profession and will gladly have you follow them around.

THE MORE HANDS-ON MEDICAL EXPERIENCE YOU HAVE, THE STRONGER YOU WILL BE AS A CANDIDATE.

MANY APPLICANTS VIEW PA SCHOOL AS A STEPPING-STONE TO MEDICAL SCHOOL. THIS IS A HUGE MISTAKE.

MATURITY

The mean age of a PA is 42. However, the maturity we look for in an applicant doesn't necessarily have anything to do with age. The committee member reviewing your application is well aware that you will likely have a patient's life in your hands on any given day. You must demonstrate maturity through your prior work experience, in your essay, and at the interview. Some basic questions the committee will want answered include:

Can you be empathetic, yet assertive?
Can you handle stress under fire?
Will you know when to call for help?
Do you exhibit good judgment?
Can you make quick decisions?
Are you a self-starter?
Will you require constant supervision?

Don't assume these questions are relative to medical experience only. PA school applicants come from diverse backgrounds and possess a variety of life experiences. Some of the most interesting candidates have careers that are totally unrelated to health care at the time of application. A typical applicant pool may have an attorney, a school-teacher, and an actress among its ranks. Ages may range from 21 to sixty-one. The common trait that most mature applicants share is the ability to exhibit a youthful energy coupled with practical life experience.

Now that you have a better understanding of exactly what the committee looks for in an applicant, let's see if we can come up with a specific plan for achieving this worthy goal.

YOU MUST DEMONSTRATE MATURITY THROUGH YOUR PRIOR WORK EXPERIENCE, IN YOUR ESSAY, AND AT THE INTERVIEW.

Getting into the
PA SCHOOL
of Your Choice

Getting into the
PA SCHOOL
of Your Choice

Setting Goals

3

> Whatever the mind of man can conceive and believe, it can achieve.
>
> —*Napoleon Hill*

WHY SET GOALS?

Few people bother to set realistic goals in life. Most people are what Zig Ziglar calls in his video, *Goals, Setting and Achieving Them on Schedule*, "a wandering generality," when they need to become "a meaningful specific." The bottom line is that the competition for getting into PA school is fierce. Without a written goal, a plan of action, and the ability to focus, your chances of being accepted to the program of your choice are slim.

The basic problem most people have with setting goals is not time, but rather a lack of direction. Everyone has the same twenty-four hours to work with each day. Why is it that some people who are intelligent and capable achieve so much, while others who are equally so can't seem to get anything accomplished? The former have goals—written, measurable, and realistic— and they know how to achieve them. Numerous authors, from Stephen Covey to Norman Vincent Peale, have discussed how to go about goal-setting. They agree that specific long- and short-range goals will lead you to become more creative, which will, in turn, add more excitement and fulfillment to your life.

Do you know why 97% of people never really set goals in the proper fashion? As Zig Ziglar says, the answer is **FEAR,** or False Evidence Appearing Real. But what are we afraid of? Some of us are afraid of failure. Some of us fear the competition. Some of us are afraid of success. After all, there is danger in setting goals; we might actually achieve them! We've all heard the phrase *Be careful what you pray for, you just might get it.*

However, there is also danger in not setting goals—the danger of wasting your resources; *a boat in dry-dock rots quicker than a boat at sea.* Don't waste your natural resources; write down your goals today. (See Appendix C.)

If I haven't yet convinced you of the importance of goal-setting, perhaps this next story will. In 1953, a study at Yale University polled the graduating seniors with respect to how many of them had written goals and a plan of action for carrying them out. Surprisingly, only 3% of these Ivy Leaguers bothered to take the steps necessary to achieve their goals. Only 10%

WITHOUT A WRITTEN GOAL, A PLAN OF ACTION, AND THE ABILITY TO FOCUS, YOUR CHANCES OF BEING ACCEPTED TO THE PROGRAM OF YOUR CHOICE ARE SLIM.

took some of the steps, and 87 % set no goals at all and had no plan of action for life after graduation—*wandering generalities*.

In 1973, those same graduating seniors were re-polled in areas that were considered measurable: finances, career, and position in life. Not surprisingly, those 3% of graduates who had set goals and had written a plan of action to carry them out accomplished more than the other 97% of graduates combined.

SEVEN-STEP FORMULA FOR SUCCESS

If you learn this seven-step formula for success, it won't make a difference what the goal is, you will be able to accomplish it. By knowing and following these seven steps you will maximize your chances of getting into the PA school of your choice.

Step 1. Identify the goal
Step 2. Set a deadline for achievement
Step 3. List obstacles to overcome
Step 4. Identify people and organizations that can help you
Step 5. List the skills and knowledge required to achieve your goal
Step 6. Develop a plan of action
Step 7. List the benefits of achieving the goal; ask yourself, *What's in it for me?*

Now what I would like you to do is to take out your pencil and paper and begin listing your goals. If you do nothing else with this book, I'll consider this one action step a success if you complete your goal sheet. If you need some help getting started, take a look below at my written goal statement for getting into PA school for 1992. (You will notice that I wrote out my goals in paragraph form. You can write your goals however you prefer. The point is to get started with the writing.)

August 15, 1990

By May 1, 1992 I will be accepted into Yale, University of Florida, or Bowman Gray's Physician Assistant Program. In order to accomplish this goal, I will first have to discuss my desire to become a PA with my wife and convince her that this is the right thing to do for our family. Next, I will need to begin saving money so that I can help my wife support our two children and provide food and shelter for the next two years. Finally, I will stay focused and not listen to those people who will say I'm "crazy" or having an "early mid-life crisis" for wanting to quit a great job at age 35 and go back to school for two years.

I will immediately contact the American Academy of Physician Assistants (AAPA) and the Connecticut Academy of Physician Assistants (ConnAPA) to find out what resources are available to me. I will get a PA Programs Directory and begin writing to several schools, focusing on my top three choices. I will contact the president of ConnAPA and get to know him. I will also visit Yale's PA program and visit with Elaine Grant, who is the Dean of the program, and maintain contact with her quarterly. I will do the same thing at the other two programs. I will find out from these people what I lack as a competitive candidate and how I can best strengthen my application.

I will visit with some PAs who work in my wife's office and spend as much time with them as possible (shadowing). I will attend as many open houses as possible to learn more about each program and to make myself known to them.

I will need Anatomy and Physiology (I & II) and Microbiology to fulfill requirements (prerequisites). I will achieve no less than an A in each class. I will also begin volunteering at Saint Raphael's hospital, in the ER, in order to gain more "current" experience. I will also obtain an SAT study guide to prepare myself for the test, which I need to take to get into Yale.

My plan is to continue working full time, save money, and do volunteer work part time. I will also take evening classes. While working in a hospital, I will discuss my goals with as many PAs as possible and learn as much as I can about the PA profession.

Once I achieve my goal of getting into the PA school of my choice, I will enjoy many benefits: helping people, job satisfaction, secure future, challenging work, stimulating work, prestige, a sense of accomplishment, and much more.

I wrote these goals in 1990. I can also vividly remember the exact moment I decided to apply to PA school. I was on vacation with my family in Orlando, Florida. I was in the office of my friend, Chuck Ruotolo, looking through the classifieds when I spotted a job opening for a Plastic Surgery PA. On a whim, I called the number and spoke with the office secretary. She practically begged me to come in for an interview. In my excitement, I forgot to tell her that I wasn't a PA at all, but I didn't want to spoil her enthusiasm. It was at that exact moment that I told my friend Chuck I was going to become a PA. He said "Go for it" and I have never looked back.

Twelve years later, as I sit writing the second edition to this book and after being a practicing PA for over eight years, I recognize that moment as one of the turning points in my life. I have never regretted my decision to become a PA. I've enjoyed all of the benefits I listed on my goal sheet above, and much more than I could have dreamed of.

Here's another example of an applicant who, having put a hurried application together for PA school and failed to get in, reassessed his priorities and concentrated on new goals.

I planned for things to be different next year. I would:

▶ Identify schools I could apply to using the Association of PA Programs (APAP) directory of PA programs
▶ Apply to at least five new schools to increase the opportunity of being interviewed
▶ Request and complete a school's application as soon as it was available
▶ Type and proofread everything I sent to the program
▶ Join the AAPA as an affiliate member
▶ Visit as many programs as I could during a summer trip East
▶ Continue to take classes that would prepare me for PA school

By the end of the year I had applied to nine schools. I had attended one interview and had three more after the first year. To prepare for these, I read several interview books and bought a new suit. I studied up on some of the issues facing the profession and health care in general. I tried to relax. The interviews were similar in format, as were the questions. Then I had to wait. Two weeks after the last interview, I was notified by my top choice that I was accepted. The years of going to school during the day and working at night, the preparation for the interviews, and the trips across the country had all paid off. I was in.

—*George Brothers, PA-C*

IMAGING

This brings me to another topic that I would like to discuss with you; it's called *imaging*. Imaging is a technique that I learned in Officer's Training

School (OTS) while becoming an officer in the U.S. Air Force. It's a powerful tool. You may be familiar with the quote at the beginning of this chapter, *Whatever the mind of man can conceive and believe, it can achieve.* This is a true statement. Try to get a crystal-clear image of yourself performing well at the interview, calm and relaxed. Picture yourself going to the mailbox and opening that acceptance letter. Each day spend a little time thinking about your goal until it becomes an obsession. You'll be surprised at the results. I used to spend a half-hour per day on my exercise machine visualizing my goal. I had a perfect image of the acceptance letter, down to the color of the school's logo. I would get myself worked up into a frenzy just thinking about it. I calculated that I spent about 180 hours imaging.

Guess what? My efforts paid off. I interviewed at the University of Florida in December 1991, on a Friday. The next Monday I received a phone call from the program congratulating me on my acceptance. I also got accepted to Yale's program in March 1992. I chose to stay local and go to Yale. I also received an invitation to interview at Bowman Gray in North Carolina. I achieved my goal of getting into the PA school of my choice (Yale) by having a written goal, working hard, and by simply carrying out my written plan of action.

> I ACHIEVED MY GOAL OF GETTING INTO THE PA SCHOOL OF MY CHOICE (YALE) BY HAVING A WRITTEN GOAL, WORKING HARD, AND BY SIMPLY CARRYING OUT MY WRITTEN PLAN OF ACTION.

TAKE A PERSONAL EVALUATION

Periodically, you must review your performance and evaluate those areas in which you need improvement; a personal inventory, if you will. Look at these seven specific areas:

1. Appearance
2. Family
3. Financial
4. Social
5. Spiritual
6. Mental
7. Career

Every so often evaluate yourself with respect to the above areas and ask yourself questions like:

- ▶ Do I present myself well? Do I need to lose some weight or buy a new pair of shoes for the interview?
- ▶ Is my family supportive of my goal? Will this career change cause conflict in my family life? Am I willing to listen to the skeptics, or follow my dream unconditionally?
- ▶ Can I afford to go to PA school now? Does the school offer graduate level student loans? Can I save enough money between now and the time school starts?
- ▶ Am I a team player? Am I willing to practice medicine as a "dependent" practitioner?
- ▶ Is it morally right for me to do this now? Do I have other obligations or responsibilities? Am I being selfish?
- ▶ Should I take any additional courses, or retake any courses? Am I well read on medical issues and current events? Will I have many distractions?
- ▶ Do I really know why I want to become a PA, versus a physician or nurse practitioner? Do I fully understand the role of the PA?

Score your answers in these seven areas on a scale from 1 to 5, with 5 being the highest and 1 being the lowest. Be honest with yourself. Work on those areas in which you score low. Taking this personal inventory will keep you focused and help you reach your goals that much quicker.

SET BIG GOALS

There were once two men fishing on a pier; one old and one young. The young man watched as the older man kept reeling in big fish but throwing them back into the water. "Why are you throwing back those big, beautiful fish?" asked the young man. "Because I only have this little frying pan," replied the old man, holding up a scrawny little skillet.

The point is to set big goals and go for the gold! Dig down deep into your soul and focus on what you want in life. Make a plan and see yourself accomplishing each task. Emerson once wrote, "What lies behind us and what lies in front of us, pales in significance to what lies within us."

WHO DO I SHARE MY GOALS WITH?

The rule is that you share *give up* goals with everybody and *go up* goals only with the people you love and trust to support your efforts. For example, if you want to lose twenty pounds, a *give up* goal, let everybody at home and at the office know about it. In contrast, if your goal is to get into PA school, a *go up* goal, share only with your closest friends and family who will tend to support you.

GETTING FOCUSED

Before leaving this chapter, I would like to touch on the power of focus. Just because you've decided to apply to PA school does not mean that *life* stops happening. You are still going to have to deal with the daily stressors that life throws your way, like finding enough time to research schools and fill out applications, taking additional courses (if necessary), balancing your business and family life, and managing financial pressures. Some applicants may find it too overwhelming to deal with all of these issues and decide to throw in the towel. Before you find yourself in this position, know that it is absolutely normal to feel overwhelmed at times. All of us have felt the same way. In fact, I felt overwhelmed a lot during PA school, but I learned some techniques that helped me to survive, and thrive. I would like to pass on one of those techniques with you right now.

List Your Top 25 Goals

In this chapter, I asked you to consider setting goals in seven specific areas: appearance, family, financial, social, spiritual, mental, and career. Since this book is about getting into PA school, I will focus on career goals, specifically as they relate to applying to PA school. Keep in mind, however, that this technique I am about to share with you will work for all seven areas above.

The first thing to do is list 25 goals, right off the top of your head, that you need to accomplish in order to be a strong applicant for PA school. To do this properly, you will need the brochures and information on each of the schools you are applying to. Write down *everything* you will need to do, in no particular order. For example, if you plan to apply to PA school in one year, your list may look like this:

1. Prepare for SATs
2. Take SATs
3. Take microbiology course at local college
4. Find three PAs to shadow
5. Gain one more year of hands-on experience
6. Start working on essay
7. Locate three people who will write a letter of reference for me
8. Join the AAPA as an affiliate member
9. Join my state chapter of the AAPA as an affiliate member
10. Save $50 per week to augment my income while in school
11. Locate and speak with three graduate PAs from the schools I am applying to
12. Attend each school's open house
13. Schedule a phone conversation with each school's director
14. Request applications from each school I am applying to
15. Find out dates SATs are given
16. Register for microbiology class
17. Contact volunteer offices at local hospitals
18. Fill out applications
19. Send for college transcripts and send to each PA program
20. Learn about the history of each program that I am applying to
21. Buy a new suit for the interview
22. Create a file for each program with application deadlines on the cover
23. Attend a meeting of the state chapter of the AAPA
24. Search the Internet for sites relevant to PA school applicants
25. Be able to talk about five current issues facing the PA profession

If you can list more than 25 goals, by all means, please do so. I know that the list can look overwhelming at times. Relax, I am going to show you how to prioritize your list and make it very manageable.

Prioritize the List

Now that you have listed everything you need to do before you become a strong PA school applicant, the next step is to prioritize. Take a look at each one of your 25 goals and determine a realistic time frame for accomplishment.

Beside each goal write a number—3, 6, 9, or 12 months. This will give you a general timeframe to work from. For example, if you need to take the SATs before you apply to PA school, you will probably place a 3 next to goal #15, *Find out dates SATs are given*, because you may want to take the SATs twice in order to maximize your score. You will also want to be sure that you have plenty of time to take the SATs and get the scores to the appropriate PA programs before their application deadline. On the other hand, you will probably place a 12 next to goal #21, since buying a new suit for the interview is likely to be one of the last things you'll need to do.

The "NCAA Tournament Draw"

The next step is to list all of your 3s on the left-hand side of a clean sheet of paper. As an example, I chose eight 3s from the above list as follows:

1. Prepare for SATs
2. Take SATs
3. Join AAPA
4. Join state chapter of AAPA
5. Save $50 per week
6. Request applications from PA schools
7. Find out SAT test dates
8. Register for microbiology class

Now place these goals in format similar to what newspapers publish during the NCAA basketball tournament in March of each year.

	ROUND 1	ROUND 2	ROUND 3	WINNER
1.	Take SATs			
		Find out SAT test dates		
2.	Find out SAT test dates		Find out SAT test dates	
3.	Join AAPA			
		Join state chapter of AAPA		
4.	Join state chapter of AAPA			
5.	Save $50 per week			Register for micro-biology course
		Request PA school applications		
6.	Request PA school applications		Register for micro-biology course	
7.	Prepare for SATs	Register for micro-biology course		
8.	Register for micro-biology course			

Instead of placing eight college basketball teams in the left-hand column, you are substituting your 3-month goals for getting into PA school. Then, **you** decide which goal moves on to the next "round" based on the significance you place on that goal versus the others. In our example, registering for a microbiology class wins out because there may be only two semesters in which you can take this course. If you do not complete this course prior to the PA school's application deadline, you probably won't have a chance of getting accepted. Therefore, by the process of elimination, I would choose registering for a microbiology class as my number-one goal to accomplish in the next three months.

Once you accomplish your number-one priority (goal), you can work backwards until all of your 3-month goals are accomplished. You can make up a similar format for your 6-, 9-, and 12-month goals. By following this format for each time frame, you will be able to stay focused on your top priorities. You will also eliminate the frustration and chaos that sometimes overwhelms us when we don't know what to do next.

The take home message in this chapter is to set big goals, write them down, follow the seven-step formula for success, and use the NCAA tournament draw method to prioritize your list and help you focus.

Selecting a Program

4

It is your work in life that is the ultimate seduction.

—*Pablo Picasso*

All physician assistant programs are not created equally. Many programs have a primary care focus, while a few have a surgical focus. Many programs offer a master's degree, while others offer a graduate certificate, bachelor's degree, or an associate's degree. Most programs average two years in length, but some are longer. Tuition varies from a few thousand dollars at some programs to over $20,000 at others. Some programs are affiliated with a medical school, while others are not. Some programs favor applicants from their home state. Why spend a great deal of energy and money applying to a particular school only to find out later that you aren't really a good fit for that particular program? In this chapter, I will give you some food for thought to consider before you apply to any given program.

At this time I would like to encourage you, once again, to join the American Academy of Physician Assistants (AAPA) as an affiliate member, and your state chapter affiliate of the AAPA. To join the AAPA call or write:

The American Academy of Physician Assistants
950 N. Washington Street
Alexandria, VA 22314-1552
Phone: (703) 836-2272
Fax: (703) 684-1924
Email: aapa@aapa.org
Web: www.aapa.org/

To join your state chapter, see Appendix E.

ACCREDITATION

Your first order of business, when deciding on which program(s) you want to apply to, is to consider the accreditation status of the program. You want to attend a program that is accredited by the Commission on Accreditation of Allied Health Education Programs (CAAHEP). The Accreditation Review Committee on Education for the Physician Assistant (ARC-PA) includes representatives from the American Medical Association (AMA), the Association of Physician Assistant Programs (APAP), the American Academy of Family Physicians, the American Academy of Pediatrics, the American College of Physicians, and the American College of Surgeons. As of this writing, there are 136 accredited PA programs.

If you do not graduate from an accredited PA program, you will not be eligible to sit for the national certifying examination for physician assistants, which is administered by the National Commission on Certification of Physician Assistants (NCCPA). Without your NCCPA certification, you will not be eligible for state licensure and you won't be able to practice medicine in most locations.

If you are applying to a relatively new program, check to make sure that it has a *provisional accreditation* status, which means it has received a comprehensive evaluation prior to opening. Although having this evaluation does not guarantee automatic accreditation, at least you can get an idea of where the program stands in the accreditation process.

If you have any questions or concerns relative to accreditation issues, contact:

> Accreditation Review Committee on Education for the Physician
>   Assistant
> 1000 North Oak Avenue
> Marshfield, WI 54449-5788
> (715) 389-3785

FOCUS OF THE PROGRAM

Most admissions committees select applicants based on several criteria that include, but are not limited to: academics, test scores (SAT, GRE, AHPAT, TOEFL, etc.), understanding of the PA profession and concept, health care experience, volunteer work, community service, interviews, the narrative statement (essay), and references. Certain programs, however, will mention in their selection criteria that the program has a particular focus: primary care, in-state residents, surgical, etc. It is important to know the focus of various programs in order to apply to those that seem to be the best fit for your qualifications and goals.

The following is a listing of PA programs that specifically mention *key words* in the *Selection Factors* section of their application or brochure. The reader should keep in mind that these factors are not always absolute criteria, and the applicant should always consult with the individual programs to get an idea of the significance of each one.

Practice in Under-served Areas

> Charles R. Drew University of Medicine and Science
> University at California, Davis
> Stanford University
> University of Southern California School of Medicine—"recruiting
>   disadvantaged applicants"
> George Washington University—"recruiting disadvantaged applicants"
> Emory University School of Medicine
> Augsburg College
> City University of New York/Harlem Hospital Center
> University of North Dakota School of Medicine

Oregon Health Sciences University
Philadelphia College of Textiles and Science
University of Utah School of Medicine

State Residents Receive Preference

Charles R. Drew University of Medicine and Science
Medical College of Georgia
Cook County Hospital/Malcolm X College
Wichita State University
University of South Dakota (tri-state: NE Nebraska, NW Iowa, and
    SE South Dakota)
Oregon Health Sciences University
Bowman Gray School of Medicine of Wake Forest
The University of Texas Medical Branch
University of Utah School of Medicine (intermountain west region)

Primary Care

Emory University School of Medicine
Albany-Hudson
Bayley-Seton Hospital
Oregon Health Sciences University

Surgeon Assitant Programs

University of Alabama at Birmingham
Cornell University Medical College
Cuyahoga Community College

Nursing Background

University of North Dakota School of Medicine

Physician Preceptor

University of California, Davis

Test Scores

University of Colorado School of Medicine
King's College

Well-defined Goals

Touro College of Health Sciences
Kettering College of Medical Arts

Christian Service

Trevecca Nazarene University

Fluency in Spanish

The University of Texas Medical Branch

Do not become discouraged or intimidated by the above list. For example, I personally know of several George Washington University graduates who were neither *disadvantaged* nor working in *under-served* areas. I once interviewed a graduate of North Dakota's PA program for a cardiothoracic surgery position. There are plenty of exceptions to most of the programs listed above. No program is going to force you to work in a particular state or in a particular specialty. There is nothing to stop a graduate of one of the surgeon assistant programs from working in primary care after graduation. The reason I list these programs and their preferences is to give you an idea as to what the admissions committee may key in on.

THE EDUCATIONAL EXPERIENCE

Before we get to the issue of master's versus bachelor's programs, let's examine some other aspects of a program that may be just as important to you and your educational experience.

It is important to remember that as long as you attend an accredited PA program you are eligible to sit for the national boards. If you pass the boards, you can work as a PA. For some of us, that may good enough. However, the quality of the individual PA program may be a deciding factor on whether you apply to one school versus another. For instance, some programs teach anatomy using cadavers, while other programs use plastic models and slides. Some programs are affiliated with a medical school and enjoy the benefits and facilities that go with it, while others are located at a four-year college or a community college. Some programs are taught by MD residents and fellows, while others are taught by PAs. Finally, some programs cost over $20,000 to attend versus other programs that cost a fraction of that amount. Only you can decide on what is most important to your educational experience.

MASTER'S VERSUS BACHELOR'S

One of the most frequently asked questions I get from prospective PA students is, "Does it matter if you have a bachelor's degree versus a master's degree to work as a PA?" The answer used to be a definitive No. However, the trend in PA education is certainly headed toward more master's programs. Many feel it's time for PA education to reach this graduate level. In 1997, a little less than 8% of PA school graduates earned a master's degree from their respective programs. In 2002, that number is expected to reach just over twenty percent.

Despite a shift toward master's programs, having a graduate degree still has no effect on whether you will get a job after graduation. It will probably be several years before having a master's degree has any effect on the marketplace at all.

On the other hand, if you get accepted into a program that offers a master's degree and one that doesn't, you may have to give the matter some additional thought. For instance, if you have aspirations to teach or become a faculty member at a PA program, you will more than likely need the master's degree. Keep in mind, though, that programs that offer a master's degree tend to cost much more in tuition expenses than those that offer a certificate or a bachelor's degree. If you don't plan to teach or become a faculty member, you may never recoup this difference financially. In addition, there are now many programs that offer PAs the opportunity to get a master's on-

ONE OF THE MOST FREQUENTLY ASKED QUESTIONS I GET FROM PROSPECTIVE PA STUDENTS IS,"DOES IT MATTER IF YOU HAVE A BACHELOR'S DEGREE VERSUS A MASTER'S DEGREE TO WORK AS A PA?" THE ANSWER USED TO BE A DEFINITIVE NO. HOWEVER, THE TREND IN PA EDUCATION IS CERTAINLY HEADED TOWARD MORE MASTER'S PROGRAMS.

line, after they graduate from PA school. Some of these programs are fairly inexpensive, yet provide the same credentials as the more expensive PA programs.

PASS/FAIL RATE

More important than which degree or certificate a PA program offers is the program's **first-time pass/fail rate** on the national boards. If only 50% of a program's graduates pass the national certifying examination on the first try, the significance of your master's degree may not be so paramount. When considering various programs, be sure to inquire about the first-time pass/fail rate on the boards. I stress *first-time* because many programs may simply give you the *overall* pass/fail rate, meaning eventually 90% of graduates pass the boards. You should also be aware of the fact that once you've already failed the boards, your odds of passing them the next time decrease significantly each time you sit for the exam.

OTHER ISSUES TO CONSIDER

I have already covered some of the main issues to consider when selecting a program; now let's look at some other factors that may influence your decision.

Clinical Rotations

Once you complete your didactic training, you will embark on your clinical rotations, where you will learn and practice your clinical skills. You will learn to take a thorough medical history and complete a comprehensive physical examination on real patients. You will be required to adapt to various preceptors and the intricacies of each facility you work in. You will find that as soon as you begin to get comfortable at one site and learn where all the bathrooms and cafeteria are located, it will be time to move on to your next rotation.

Clinical rotations provide you with an opportunity to grow as a clinician. It is important that the schools you consider have well-established clinical rotation sites that provide a rewarding experience for the student. Most schools have mandatory clinical rotations in family practice, internal medicine, surgery, emergency room, pediatrics, obstetrics and gynecology, and psychiatry. In addition, students can pick from a variety of elective rotations. Since you are the one paying for your education, be sure you get the most for your dollar.

Another suggestion is to talk with the students at the various programs. Find out what they like and dislike about their clinical experience. Ask about the ratio of medical students to PA students on any given rotation. Are PA students given the same opportunities as the medical students, or are they lower on the food chain? Many programs keep a running file on the various rotation sites, with written feedback from students after completing the rotation. Ask if you can read some of these comments, since students tend to comment on everything, from the quality of the clinical experience to parking and accommodations. This is valuable information and will serve to guide you when it's time for you to select a program and/or rotation sites when you are a student.

WHEN CONSIDERING VARIOUS PROGRAMS, BE SURE TO INQUIRE ABOUT THE FIRST-TIME PASS/FAIL RATE ON THE BOARDS.

CLINICAL ROTATIONS PROVIDE YOU WITH AN OPPORTUNITY TO GROW AS A CLINICIAN. IT IS IMPORTANT THAT THE SCHOOLS YOU CONSIDER HAVE WELL-ESTABLISHED CLINICAL ROTATION SITES THAT PROVIDE A REWARDING EXPERIENCE FOR THE STUDENT.

Parking and Housing

How will you get to school every day? Can you afford to pay the going rate for rent in the city or town where you will attend school? You must consider these issues before you decide on any given program. Take into account the cost of living, parking, food, utilities, etc. A good place to start your research is with the Chamber of Commerce, which will gladly mail you enough literature to make an informed decision.

MORE TIPS

The following is a short list of tips that may aid you in the decision-making process. If you follow all of these suggestions, you will be a well-informed applicant. Applicants who do their homework tend to perform well at the interview.

Order the PA Programs Directory

The PA School Programs Directory is offered exclusively by the Association of Physician Assistant Programs (APAP). The directory lists all of the accredited PA programs in the United States. It also includes information on tuition, prerequisites, financial aid, tests scores, essay requirements and content, curriculum, and clinical rotations. The directory is no longer published in a book format, but can be purchased on-line through APAP at: www.apap.org/directory/index.htm.

Attend the Open House

Attending a program's open house is a must if you are serious about the program. First of all, it gives the program an opportunity to match your face with your name. Most programs also keep a record of open house attendees, which may eventually help your overall score on your application.

Next, attending the open house gives you insight into the program. By listening to the program speakers you can get a good feel for the philosophy of the program, which can be helpful when writing your essay or interviewing. You also have the opportunity to meet some of the current students and faculty. **You may even chat with someone who'll be interviewing you later.** Of course, attending the open house doesn't guarantee you an interview, but in this highly competitive environment it certainly won't hurt your chances either.

In addition, you have the opportunity to meet and size up the competition. By speaking with other applicants, especially those who may have interviewed elsewhere, you may get some ideas on ways to strengthen your application. Take this opportunity to soak up as much information as you can from everyone that you meet that day.

Finally, after attending the open house you may decide that a particular school is not a good fit for you. Perhaps you are not impressed with the faculty or the quality of the students. Maybe the program appears to be unorganized, which is not uncommon with newer programs. In any case, it is better that you find this out as soon as possible, before you accept a position in a particular class.

Speak with the Program Director

Whether you attend the open house or not, speak to the school's program director at least once before you apply. If you live nearby or plan on visiting the area, set up a face-to-face appointment. Again, this is an opportunity to allow someone on the admissions committee to place a face with your name. If you do get an interview with the program director, be sure to dress appropriately and have a list of relevant questions prepared prior to the meeting. Remember, each encounter that you have with program faculty is evaluated in one way or another; be sure your encounter is a positive one.

Visit Local Hospitals or Clinics

Stop by the local hospital or clinic and see how many of the program's graduates are employed there. Ask the physicians and nurses how they feel about the PAs who work there, especially the graduates of the program you are interested in. Does the PA school have a good reputation in the community? While visiting the facility, speak to some of the graduate PAs who now work there and ask them if they are happy with the education they received at the program. By the time you leave you will have a good idea as to the quality of the program.

WHETHER YOU ATTEND THE OPEN HOUSE OR NOT, SPEAK TO THE SCHOOL'S PROGRAM DIRECTOR AT LEAST ONCE BEFORE YOU APPLY.

Completing the Application

5

In this chapter, I will discuss the procedures for completing the PA school application. I include all of the components that must be delivered to the admissions committee in order to be considered for an interview. Some schools may require that you fill out two separate applications: one application for the PA program and one for the college or university itself. The latter is usually a formality if you meet all of the requirements of the PA program. I discuss the application process, and how candidates are scored and selected for interview. I also touch on the letter of recommendation, pointing out whom you should obtain letters from, what the letters should say, and how to obtain the perfect letter of reference. Finally, I will provide detailed information on the relatively new Central Application Service for Physician Assistants (CASPA).

Most applications require the following items:

- ▶ Application fee
- ▶ Application form(s)
- ▶ Test Scores (SAT/ACT, GRE, AHPAT, TOEFL, etc.)
- ▶ Transcripts (college and high school)
- ▶ Three evaluation (reference) letters
- ▶ U.S. Government form DD214 (applicable for veterans)
- ▶ Professional certificates
- ▶ Narrative statement (essay)

If you are reapplying to a program, you should re-do all of the forms again, including the essay. Hopefully, you will be able to favorably update last year's application and present even more evidence that the committee should select you this time.

Each school has its own requirements for admission. The key, on any application, is to **pay strict attention to detail,** accomplish the forms as soon as possible, and send for your transcripts early enough to meet the various program deadlines. In addition, be sure that you meet the program's prerequisite requirements before you apply, or that you are at least enrolled in a prerequisite class at the time of application. Let the program know if you are currently enrolled in a prerequisite class so they know you will be a fully qualified candidate by the program start date. Occasionally, a program may waive a particular prerequisite based on your prior experience or circumstances. Always get any waiver in writing.

THE KEY, ON ANY APPLICATION, IS TO PAY STRICT ATTENTION TO DETAIL.

A professional application should be typed, unless otherwise instructed, and error-free. This means no spelling errors, typos, etc. A great way to check your application for spelling errors is to read the entire application backwards. This may take some time to do, but the results are well worth it. You'll find that by reading the text backwards, spelling errors will pop right out of the page. I also recommend that you have at least one other person read your application for errors and overall content.

Spelling errors can be the kiss of death for an applicant. If you aren't capable of paying strict attention to detail on a graduate level application, how can the committee trust that you will focus on the details of your patients? Will you also miss a critical lab value, or a fracture on a child's x-ray? The point is clear; your application can speak volumes about you before the committee even gets to meet you.

THE APPLICATION PROCESS

The typical PA program is approximately two years in length, full time. A few programs are three or four years in length. Application deadlines vary for each program; however, a general rule is that applications are due between September and January for classes entering the following summer or fall. If you are applying to a program with *rolling admissions* you can submit your application at any time; however, if you do not apply early enough you may be *rolling over* until the next year, since it's first come, first served at these schools. Most programs interview students in January and February, so give the committee plenty of time to give your application a fair evaluation.

The application review process is complex, yet comprehensive. There exists an extensive set of checks and balances to ensure that the best candidates are interviewed. There are several committee members involved in each application, so your fate is not controlled by any single person. Let's take a look at the process and see how a successful candidate navigates his/her way through the system. Please keep in mind that the following procedure is from a *typical* program; each school may evaluate its applicants however it wishes.

Initially, once you have completed the application and submitted all of the supporting material, the program registrar checks your file for completeness, organizes the file, and passes it on for admissions committee review.

Most programs have several volunteers who sit on the admissions committee, evaluate applications, and conduct applicant interviews. The committee is comprised of program faculty, program PA students, graduate PAs who work in the community, and various other medical professionals.

Each committee member is issued a stack of applications to review and score. That same stack of applications is then passed on to two other committee members for review and scoring. Usually, the records are reviewed by male and female committee members. In giving you a score, the committee member considers your medical experience, narrative statement (essay), references, work history, and your understanding of the PA profession. There is no particular factor that influences your overall score more than any other; however, a poorly written essay or a less than desirable letter of recommendation can certainly ruin your chances of getting an invitation to interview.

Once all of the applicants receive a score, the committee meets to select a group of applicants to interview. The number of applicants who get in-

SPELLING ERRORS CAN BE THE KISS OF DEATH FOR AN APPLICANT.

THERE IS NO PARTICULAR FACTOR THAT INFLUENCES YOUR OVERALL SCORE MORE THAN ANY OTHER; HOWEVER, A POORLY WRITTEN ESSAY OR A LESS THAN DESIRABLE LETTER OF RECOMMENDATION CAN CERTAINLY RUIN YOUR CHANCES OF GETTING AN INVITATION TO INTERVIEW.

vited to interview will vary from program to program. Many schools, however, will interview approximately 100 applicants per year.

Selecting these 100 candidates for an interview involves one final process. After tallying the scores of each candidate, the committee will usually unanimously agree on 75 or so applicants who are clearly and objectively the cream of the crop. It is the selection of the remaining 25 applicants that makes the interview selection process so interesting and sometimes controversial. One committee member may make a very strong case for a particular candidate, while two other members may argue strongly against that same applicant. Sometimes a spelling error or a poor letter of reference can be the difference between getting accepted and getting rejected.

After the smoke clears and the final cut is made, many committee members ponder over those applicants who were turned down because of spelling errors or a poorly written essay. As a committee member, you always wonder if you've made the right choices or perhaps let a great prospect slip through the cracks.

In any event, as an applicant, make sure that your application is error-free and your essay is well written. This way you're sure to be evaluated on your strengths rather than your weaknesses.

LETTERS OF RECOMMENDATION

As part of the application process, you are required to provide at least three letters of recommendation in support of your application. Be sure to pay strict attention to detail relative to each school's specific requirements for references. For instance, some schools may allow you to choose your own personal references. Other programs specify that you should have letters from a PA, a physician, and a former supervisor.

When you are considering potential candidates who will provide you with a great letter of reference, **be sure to include at least one PA.** After all, you are applying to a PA program, and the committee would like to know that you've impressed another PA significantly enough to support your application. The PA profession is relatively small, and most of us (PAs) would not co-sign a potential student's application if we didn't think he or she would make a great PA. To some, this rule is quite obvious; however, plenty of applicants fail to grasp this simple concept. Applicants write about shadowing or working with PAs in their essay, but then fail to obtain a reference from this valuable resource.

Many applicants are under the false impression that the bigger the name or position, the more weight the letter of reference will carry. Nothing could be further from the truth. The admissions committee is comprised of some pretty sharp people, most of whom are PAs. The committee will favor a letter from a fellow PA over some "big shot" on any given day. If you don't know any PAs, don't fret. Get busy locating some local PAs and ask to shadow them for a day or two. Most PAs will jump at the chance to help you.

Your references will usually be asked to rate you in the following areas:

- ▶ Academic Performance
- ▶ Interpersonal skills
- ▶ Maturity
- ▶ Adaptability/flexibility
- ▶ Motivation for a career as a PA

THE COMMITTEE WILL FAVOR A LETTER FROM A FELLOW PA OVER SOME "BIG SHOT" ON ANY GIVEN DAY.

In addition, the reference will be asked to provide written comments on the following:

▶ Applicant's ability to relate well with others
▶ Strengths relative to a career as a PA
▶ Weaknesses
▶ Other comments bearing on the individual applicant

Keep in mind that a good letter of recommendation has four important features:

1. It shows that the writer truly knows the individual and can comment about the applicant's qualifications.
2. It shows that the writer knows enough about the applicant and can make comparative judgments about the applicant's intellectual, academic, and professional abilities in relation to others in a similar role.
3. It provides supporting details to make the statement believable.
4. It is short, yet concise and sincere.

When it comes to obtaining great letters of recommendation, perhaps we can learn a valuable lesson from our military friends. Both enlisted and officer personnel write their own evaluations and simply present them to their supervisors for approval and signature. This is a great way to ensure that all four criteria above are met. If the supervisor (referee) does not agree with any of your comments, he/she can make changes, however this usually doesn't happen. If you are concerned that your referee is too busy to do an effective job, or maybe doesn't have the best writing skills, you can write the letter of recommendation and simply present it to him/her for evaluation and signature. (See Appendix B for sample letters of recommendation.)

Finally, **follow up** with your referee to be sure that he/she is aware of any deadlines that need to be met. Be tactful, yet assertive. Remember, this is your future at stake here and you don't want to be rejected because of a missed letter of recommendation. This is another reason why you may want to avoid the "big shot" letter of recommendation. It can be very difficult to follow up with these big shots, or they may simply be too busy to do a timely, effective job for you.

In summary, the letter of reference plays a key role in the evaluation process of your application. I encourage you, again, to obtain at least one letter of recommendation from a physician assistant. If you absolutely cannot obtain a PA reference, ask someone who knows you well and can honestly and enthusiastically support your desire to become a PA.

CENTRAL APPLICATION SERVICE FOR PHYSICIAN ASSISTANTS (CASPA)

Applicants who are applying to more than one program may elect to use the relatively new, web-based Central Application Service for Physician Assistants (CASPA). CASPA allows applicants to apply to more than one program by completing only one application. This service is easy to use, convenient, and provides the following benefits:

▶ Reduced paperwork. Applicants submit only one application, one set of transcripts, and one set of references.

FOUR IMPORTANT FEATURES OF A GOOD LETTER OF RECOMMENDATION:
1. IT SHOWS THAT THE WRITER TRULY KNOWS THE INDIVIDUAL AND CAN COMMENT ABOUT THE APPLICANT'S QUALIFICATIONS.
2. IT SHOWS THAT THE WRITER KNOWS ENOUGH ABOUT THE APPLICANT AND CAN MAKE COMPARATIVE JUDGMENTS ABOUT THE APPLICANT'S INTELLECTUAL, ACADEMIC, AND PROFESSIONAL ABILITIES IN RELATION TO OTHERS IN A SIMILAR ROLE.
3. IT PROVIDES SUPPORTING DETAILS TO MAKE THE STATEMENT BELIEVABLE.
4. IT IS SHORT, YET CONCISE AND SINCERE.

- ▶ Streamlined processing. Applicants can apply on-line or by paper.
- ▶ Ongoing support and communication with applicants. Once an applicant's account is created, he/she can view the application's status on CASPA's web site.
- ▶ Ability to apply to multiple programs. Applicants can increase their chances of acceptance by applying to several schools.

CASPA is a service provided by the Association of Physician Assistant Programs (APAP). Applicants can contact CASPA:

By telephone: (240) 497-1895 (M–F, 9–5 EST)
By email: apply@caspaonline.org
Online: https://secure.caspaonline.org/.
By mail: CASPA, PO Box 70958, Chevy Chase, MD 20813-0958

Applications typically become available on April 15th. Program deadlines vary, as do the number of programs (69) that currently accept CASPA applications. However, I anticipate that all programs will eventually use this valuable service. The list below represents those schools who participate with CASPA as of this writing. I also list the application deadlines next to each program. The reader should have all of the application material and fees to CASPA at least 30 days prior to the deadline for a particular program.

State	Program	Application Deadline
AL	University of Alabama at Birmingham	11/15
	University of Southern Alabama	11/15
AZ	Arizona School of Health Sciences	02/01
	Midwestern University Glendale	11/01
CA	Loma Linda University	01/15
	Samuel Merritt College	12/01
	University of Southern California	10/01
	Western University of Health Sciences	11/01
CO	Red Rocks Community College	01/05
CT	Quinnipiac University (Domestic students)	12/01
	Quinnipiac University (International students)	11/01
	Yale University	12/01
DC	George Washington University	10/15
FL	Barry University	01/31
	Nova Southeastern University	12/31
	University of Florida	12/01
IA	Des Moines University/Osteopathic	12/31
	University of Iowa	12/01
ID	Idaho State University	01/15
IL	Finch University of Health Sciences	12/01
	Midwestern University	1101
IN	Butler University/Clarian Health	12/01
	University of Saint Francis	12/01
KS	Wichita State University	10/01
KY	University of Kentucky	06/01
MD	University of MD/Eastern Shore	01/15
ME	University of New England	11/01
MI	Western Michigan University	12/31
MN	Augsburg College	10/15

State	Program	Application Deadline
MO	Saint Louis University	10/01
MT	Rocky Mountain College	12/01
NE	Union College	11/23
	University of Nebraska Medical Center	11/01
NM	University of St. Francis	11/15
NY	CUNY Medical School/Harlem Hospital	01/31
	Daemen College	12/15
	LeMoyne College	01/15
	Mercy College	12/01
	NY Institute of Technology	12/01
	St. Vincent Catholic Medical Center	01/31
	SUNY Stony Brook	01/15
	Touro College-Bayshore	03/01
	Cornell University/Weill Medical College	09/01
OH	Kettering College of Medical Arts	12/01
	Marietta College	12/01
	Medical College of Ohio	12/01
	The University of Findlay	12/31
OR	Oregon Health Sciences University	11/15
	Pacific University	09/15
PA	Chatham College	12/01
	Lock Haven University	12/15
	Philadelphia College of Osteopathic Medicine	12/15
	Philadelphia University	12/15
	Saint Francis University	11/30
SD	University of South Dakota	11/01
TN	Trevecca Nazarene University	11/01
TX	Baylor College of Medicine	12/01
	Texas Tech University Health Science Center	12/15
	University of Texas Medical Branch/Galveston	12/01
	University of Texas SW Medical Center	11/15
	University of North Texas Health Science Center	11/15
UT	University of Utah	11/15
VA	College of Health Sciences	01/15
	James Madison University	09/30
	Shenandoah University	12/15
WA	University of Washington (MEDEX)	11/15
WI	University of Wisconsin/LaCrosse	11/01
	University of Wisconsin/Madison	11/01
WV	Alderson-Broaddus College	01/01

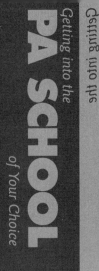
The Essay

In this chapter we cover the part of the application process that makes or breaks so many candidates: the narrative statement, or essay. Writing the essay creates a lot of stress among applicants for various reasons. Many applicants fear writing in general, and they know the essay has to be not only persuasive, but also grammatically correct to score points with the committee. Some applicants struggle with a topic, especially if one is not provided for them. Others simply don't know how to use the essay effectively to paint an accurate picture of one's self without coming off as too self-centered and arrogant.

I designed this chapter to alleviate some of the stress associated with writing your essay. I start by providing you with some suggestions on how to strengthen your essay and how to avoid some common pitfalls. I then give you five specific topics to write about, along with specific instructions for each one of them. Next, I take you through the *evolution of an essay* to show you how to develop a theme and stick with it. Finally, I provide four complete examples of *essays that worked* for others, three *annotated* essays, and some examples of essay *extracts* that demonstrate persuasive writing techniques.

Before you begin to think about writing your narrative statement (essay), take the time to fill out the worksheets at the end of this chapter. We've included several sheets so that you can gather data on your work history, medical experience, high school and college work, volunteer activities, military experience, foreign language abilities, travel experiences, and miscellaneous items. By filling out these forms before you start to write your essay, you will have organized your thoughts so that you can write a more effective essay and, in addition, perform better in your interview.

HOW IMPORTANT IS THE ESSAY?

If you were to poll 100 admissions committee members, over 90% would probably tell you that the narrative statement (essay) is the **most important** part of the application process. Fortunately, the narrative is one of the few things over which you have any control. Yes, grade point average, test scores, medical experience, and letters of recommendation are also very important, but if you fail to connect with the reader of your narrative statement, you may be passed over for an interview. Conversely, otherwise marginal candidates, with respect to test scores and grade point average, receive interviews strictly based on their very effective, emotionally charged essays.

The serious candidate spends a considerable amount of time writing and rewriting the narrative statement. She has several people read the essay for flow, content, grammar, typos, and spelling. A great technique for catching typos and spelling errors is to read your essay backwards; mistakes will jump off the page at you.

The following suggestions will help you write an effective narrative statement. Do not become frustrated if you have trouble finding the exact words at first. The key is to put the pen to the paper and *just do it*. And remember: **Under no circumstances is it acceptable to allow someone else to write your essay.**

SUGGESTIONS

1. Learn as much as you can about the program you're applying to

If you are going to spend the time, money, and effort applying to a PA program, at least attempt to learn everything you can about the school before you apply and/or interview. Study the history of the program, including the history of the university or college where it is offered. Get a feel for the philosophy of the program and the goals the program sets for educating PA students. Contact as many students and graduates of the program so you can get a good feel for the strengths and weaknesses of the program. Basically, do your homework and you'll be a much better and stronger applicant for having done so.

2. Follow instructions

Carefully read the essay question(s) and be sure your answer is relevant to the question(s) asked. Too many applicants have their own agenda; they want to tell the reader what they want to tell them instead of what is asked for. For example, if the essay question asks, How do you expect to fulfill your goals as a physician assistant?, don't write about your experiences saving lives and volunteering at the soup kitchen. Answer the question!

In addition, if the instructions call for a *two-page* narrative, do not write any more than that. In this case, more is not better. Put yourself in the committee member's place: She has already read fifty essays and now she comes across your three-pager, with size 8 font, no less. Don't give the reader of your essay any excuse for not giving it the full attention it deserves.

3. Avoid using "I" too much

In order to appear less self-centered and more team-oriented, read through your essay and limit the number of times you use the word "I." Instead, use "we," "our," and "us" more often. Give the reader the impression that you are a team player. Talk more about your patients than about yourself. I attended one open house where they told us that *if we had more than five "I"s in our essay, redo it*. This may have been stretching it just a bit, but we certainly got the point.

4. Target your audience

Remember that most committee members are physician assistants. Don't waste a lot of space in your essay writing about the duties and responsibilities of the PA. Believe it or not, many applicants use half of their essay to repeat

THE SERIOUS CANDIDATE SPENDS A CONSIDERABLE AMOUNT OF TIME WRITING AND REWRITING THE NARRATIVE STATEMENT.

I ATTENDED ONE OPEN HOUSE WHERE THEY TOLD US THAT *IF WE HAD MORE THAN FIVE "I"S IN OUR ESSAY, REDO IT.*

the AAPA definition of a physician assistant. Use this space instead to tell the reader what separates you from the other ten candidates hoping to get your interview slot.

5. Make it presentable

It goes without saying that you should type your essay on a computer and have it laser printed. If you are instructed to do otherwise, then **follow the instructions.** Do not type in small fonts; use size 12.

6. Check for spelling

Spelling errors are **inexcusable** and show a complete lack of attention to detail. The message you are sending to the committee is that you don't care enough about your application, and their program, to give your best effort. This is a sure way to be rejected for an interview. Once you finish your essay, run it through your computer's spell checker and then have someone you trust read it and provide you with feedback.

7. Organize your writing

Communicating effectively is a key part of the PA's role. If your thoughts are scattered and you cannot get organized, you will have a great deal of difficulty when it comes to explaining procedures to your patients or presenting a patient's symptoms to your attending physician on rounds.

Programs will often ask you to answer the following: *Attach to this application a typewritten narrative of not more than two pages, explaining where you learned of the PA profession, what factors or influences led you to this career choice, and how you expect to fulfill your goals as a physician associate.* Other programs will simply ask you to explain why you want to become a physician assistant. Still other programs may leave the topic up to you (more about this in the next section). Whichever situation applies to you, be sure to read the question carefully and follow directions.

TOPICS: SELECTION AND DEVELOPMENT

If you have an open-ended essay question, consider one of these topics to write about:

1. Your motivation for a career as a physician assistant.
2. The influences of your family/early experiences on your life.
3. The influence of extracurricular or work/volunteer activities on your life.
4. Your long-term goals.
5. Your personal philosophy.

Guidelines

1. Select only those topics for which you have something meaningful to say.
2. Convey your personality in your essay; make yourself appear as an interesting candidate to meet and interview.
3. Add *life* to your essay. What's important to you? What experiences had an impact on your life? What did you learn as a result of your experiences?
4. Avoid using contractions in an essay. For example, use "did not" instead of "didn't," and "I am" instead of "I'm."

5. Avoid using abbreviations in your essay unless you have used the complete term first. For example, physician assistant (PA) and emergency room (ER). In general, keep your essay more formal and avoid using abbreviations as much as possible.

6. Avoid slang or colloquial expressions. For example, instead of saying "He is a really cool professor," use "He is a great role model."

7. Avoid using run-on sentences. In other words, **keep it simple** by avoiding long sentences with excessive punctuation marks.

8. Make sure your opening paragraph is strong, well constructed, and quickly gains the attention of the reader.

9. Have a key sentence or topic sentence in each paragraph that highlights the main point of the paragraph.

10. Use vignettes, or small anecdotes as examples to back up what you say. Balance these with explanations.

11. Check the use of tenses and make sure they are consistent.

12. Avoid the use of the passive voice; it can be awkward and less effective than the active voice. For example, instead of using "The job could not be kept because . . . ," try "I could not keep the job because . . ."

13. Avoid being too wordy.

14. Conclude your essay as strongly as you began it, with a reiteration of why you want to be a PA (or what your goals are, etc.). A reiteration can add a slightly different slant to what you have already said.

MOTIVATION FOR BECOMING A PA

YOU SHOULD WRITE ABOUT YOUR MOTIVATION FOR A CAREER AS A PHYSICIAN ASSISTANT.

You should write about your motivation for a career as a physician assistant. I guarantee you that at some point during the interview they'll ask you why you want to become a PA. If you discuss this in the essay, you can deal with this question before it is asked and have a helpful outline to work with.

The first thing to do is spend some quiet time thinking about why you want to become a PA. Do some brainstorming. What experiences or people have led you to this career path? Use examples and vignettes to illustrate your point and lend credibility to your essay. The following example illustrates the point.

Although there were several excellent doctors in our pediatricians' office, we preferred using the physician assistants on our visits. The pediatricians seemed always rushed and spent little time with the physical exam; they were almost mechanical in their mannerisms. The PAs spent much more time with us and developed a special relationship with our children. They knew what sports my children were involved in, what grades they received in school, and had an overall sense of their well being. Each visit the PA would allow the children to listen to their own heartbeats, and always explained every single procedure before she performed it. I later shadowed this same PA and found out that she grew up with a lot of hardship living in a rural southern community. Yet, she had a tremendous following of patients and enjoyed every minute of her job. I believe a career as a physician assistant will allow me to work autonomously, yet collaboratively, with several members of the health care team. I'll look forward to the first time I get to hold a stethoscope up to a child's heart and ask, "Can you hear it?"

Take out a fresh sheet of paper and write this question at the top: **Why do I want to become a physician assistant?** Start brainstorming and writing down everything that comes to mind; everything goes. If you find that you are having a hard time coming up with the answers, then answer the questions below to try and focus your thoughts.

Why don't I want to become a physician?
Why don't I want to become a nurse?
Why don't I want to become a nurse practitioner?
Why don't I want to become a teacher?
Why don't I want to become a physical therapist?

Hopefully, you will now have a better understanding of why you want to become a PA. If you are still having difficulty coming up with answers, perhaps you should think hard about choosing this career path.

FAMILY/EARLY EXPERIENCES

Many applicants feel that they must write about medical experiences or educational awards to show that they have value as people. By writing about individuals or incidents that have shaped your life, you begin to paint a picture of an interesting person, someone the admissions committee would like to meet.

> I grew up one of six children. My father died when I was seven, and my mom worked two jobs to support us. She, fortunately, had an education behind her and worked as a nurse in an emergency room. I grew up with plenty of food on the table and a roof over my head, but I had very little guidance. I often got into trouble and felt lost in life. I did play a lot of sports, though, and as a result, spent numerous hours in the emergency room where my mom worked. It was here that I became fascinated with medicine. I would peek around corners to watch the doctors perform procedures on patients, and beg my mother to let me stay longer. I felt exhilarated in this environment. One day I shared my feelings with one of the residents. He made a statement which I have not forgotten to this day. He said, "Son, you can become anything you want to in life, if you only set your mind to it."
>
> As I grew older, still with no real direction in life, I often thought about those words but never totally bought into the idea. I quit high school at age sixteen with plans to join the Navy at seventeen. My mother quickly intervened, however, and arranged for me to finish high school during the summer.
>
> That summer, soon after graduation, I enlisted in the Navy and became a hospital corpsman. I grew up and matured a great deal in this environment. Most of all, however, I realized why I had such a fascination for medicine. I loved working in the collaborative environment with other health care professionals. I enjoyed providing care to my fellow servicemen and the satisfaction I felt after sewing a Marine's leg wound in the field or diagnosing an acute appendix in the clinic. For the first time in my life, I actually enjoyed waking up and going to work in the morning. I looked to the challenges that lay ahead. I became eager to learn all that I could and began taking college science courses in the evening. I did very well and began to believe that I could do anything that I set my mind to.
>
> As a result of these experiences, I feel that I have a good understanding of what it takes to provide health care. I understand the role of the physician assistant, and I would like to continue my health care experience and aspirations in this newly expanded role.

EXTRACURRICULAR ACTIVITIES AND WORK/VOLUNTEER EXPERIENCES

If you have filled out the worksheets that we provide for you at the end of this chapter, this should be an easy topic on which to write. Keep in mind

BY WRITING ABOUT INDIVIDUALS OR INCIDENTS THAT HAVE SHAPED YOUR LIFE, YOU BEGIN TO PAINT A PICTURE OF AN INTERESTING PERSON, SOMEONE THE ADMISSIONS COMMITTEE WOULD LIKE TO MEET.

that you don't always have to write about medical experiences. Show the reader what you have learned from all of your life experiences and try to demonstrate, in your writing, that you are a person of value. Don't simply repeat items (awards, honors, etc.) that you have listed on the application and that are already available to the reader.

To help you write effectively, think about answering the following questions in your writing:

1. What did you learn from your extracurricular activities or work experiences?
2. Are you a team player?
3. How have you matured as a result of your experiences?
4. If you had a leadership role, how did you contribute to getting the job done?

The key to success in this area is to lead the reader to believe, on his/her own, that you are an independent thinker and a mature person, without actually using these adjectives in your essay.

The following paragraphs, from two essays, illustrate the point I am trying to make. These writers share what they learned from volunteer and work experiences.

Sample #1

When I decided to volunteer at Saint Vincent's hospital, I felt that I had a fairly good idea of how things worked in an emergency room. After all, I worked as an emergency room technician in one of the largest hospitals in the country. What I did not know, however, was how impersonal and insensitive we can be to our patients. In my role as a patient representative I now viewed things from the other side of the fence: the patient's side. I soon realized that the staff frequently referred to the patients as the "leg" in room two or the "belly" in room five. We tell patients, "Your LFTs are elevated" but never stop to explain what "LFTs" are. We sometimes methodically examine a patient and leave her undressed, cold, and embarrassed. We don't ever bother to shut the curtain most of the time.

Since I had some medical experience, I often tried to explain the various procedures to patients and found myself frequently apologizing for the sometimes insensitive treatment. The patients really appreciated this as I received numerous letters of gratitude. Soon after starting as a volunteer I was offered a paid position in Patient Relations.

As a paid employee I found myself walking a fine line. I knew that I wanted to become a physician assistant, yet my job was mainly as a patient advocate. As a result, I often had to confront those, who may well have become my future colleagues, with patient complaints that were sometimes aimed at them. What I found was if I called patients by their names, instead of by body part, and if I quickly closed a curtain after an exam, that most of the staff started doing the same thing. This provided a much more comfortable environment for the patient and made my job a whole lot easier too.

Sample #2

Instead of joining the civilian arena after graduating from college, I decided to join the United States Air Force. I entered Officer's Training School not knowing what to expect, but with a lot of expectations. This service paid off in many ways. First, I learned to pay strict attention to detail. Second, the responsibility I had as a junior officer gave me the confidence to perform and accomplish many tasks working under less than ideal situations. Third, I learned the importance of teamwork and how to delegate responsibility in order to get the job done. Finally, I learned to always give one hundred percent since many people rely on me and trust my judgment. I left the Air Force with many accomplishments, including the Junior Officer of the Year award.

If you are a volunteer or working as a technician in the health care field, be careful not to profess that you know what it is like to be a physician assistant. On the other hand, try to let the reader know that you have thoroughly investigated the field and that you can write an intelligent and interesting essay.

IRREGULARITIES IN YOUR ACADEMIC RECORD

Most programs require you to send a copy of your college and high school transcripts with your application. Many people will have excellent academic backgrounds. Many people will also have good academic backgrounds. Some applicants, however, will have a transcript that contains a few Ds, Fs, or Ws. These people must address these grades somewhere on the application form. Some choose to use the essay itself; others will use the *additional comments* section. Choose whichever you prefer, but if you don't address this issue you may never get to the interview phase.

If you have many irregularities on your transcript, please consider retaking the classes in which you did poorly. When you write about these irregularities, **do not make excuses.** Offer an explanation as best you can without sounding as if you are a *victim* of circumstance. Point out that you are aware of the deficiencies in you record and tell the reader what you have done about it. What have you learned as a result of your mistakes?

This gentleman explains why he was suspended from school in his freshman year.

> I was accepted to Weaver College on a baseball scholarship. At the time I was used to being a "star athlete" and having everything done for me. In my freshman year I paid more attention to playing baseball, and trying to fit in with the team, than I did to my studies. As a result, my grades suffered and I was suspended for the rest of the semester. That gave me a lot of time to think about which direction I was headed in. Yes, I came to college to play baseball, but my goal was to get a good education so that I could someday fulfill my dream of working in health care. Upon returning to school that next semester I promised myself that I would change my ways and give my education top priority. I worked hard and have maintained a solid 3.3 grade point average since then. I also learned that it does not have to be all or nothing, as I continued playing baseball and volunteering at the local hospital.

The following is an example of a poor explanation for below average grades. The writer assumes no responsibility for her part in the deficiencies and this paragraph will reflect negatively on her as a mature, responsible candidate. She is what I call an "excusiologist."

> I would like to use this section of my application to write about some of the low grades I have received. I strongly feel that my transcripts do not provide an adequate representation of my ability to perform well as a physician assistant student. For example, in my sophomore year, I took organic chemistry with the same instructor for two semesters and received Ds both times. The professor and I did not hit it off very well, and I feel that he held this against me when scoring tests and lab assignments. With regards to the "F" in psychology, my entire grade was based on a paper that we had to hand in at the

end of the course. My paper was two days late because of my being away taking care of my mother who was suffering from a serious heart illness. I notified the instructor before I left that my paper might be late. I assumed that it would be all right, but when I received my grade it was too late to do anything about it. I spoke with my guidance counselor, but he informed me that the syllabus clearly states that the final paper must be handed in on time to receive a passing grade; there was nothing he could do. My attempts to contact my instructor and talk it over with her were also futile and the grade stands.

As far as the rest of the low grades are concerned, I feel as though two main factors contributed to my deficiencies. First of all, I went to a very poor high school. Many of the students were more interested in partying than studying. As a result, the teachers were frustrated and did not do a very good job trying to motivate the class. Once I got to college I had a lot of catching up to do and my grades suffered. In addition, I overloaded myself with science courses and labs in my junior year because I switched majors. I always had two or three lab reports to do per week, and this took up a great deal of my time that I would ordinarily spend studying. In my senior year, however, I really settled down and achieved a 3.5 average for the year.

This explanation is too lengthy and full of excuses. Readers of this essay are likely to put it to one side and go on to a more interesting candidate.

NONTRADITIONAL BACKGROUND

Applicants may be nontraditional by virtue of age, race, medical experience, academic background, grade point average (GPA), or life experience. Too many applicants feel that they are at a disadvantage because of this. In reality, however, a student from a nontraditional background is sometimes a more interesting candidate than the traditional applicant. It all depends on how you present yourself, and your story, to the reader. You must learn to turn your own particular situation into a positive experience.

The following excerpt is from a young woman who explains how her degree in dance and her work in massage therapy qualify her as a strong candidate.

> Through my degree in dance/kinesiology I learned of the many intricate movements the human body is capable of performing, as well as the limitations of our muscles, bones, and joints. Soon after graduating I opened a small practice as a massage therapist. I worked with a variety of patients and found that my best skill was listening intently to complaints and spending enough time with the patient to work them out. I continued to study anatomy and physiology in order to best serve my patients. I now have a longing to do more. I would like to build on what I have learned and begin to diagnose and treat patients in the medical arena. I am confident that my prior experience will aid me in this quest.

The above writer also does a great job demonstrating that she possesses *transferable skills*. Although she has not worked directly in a clinical setting, she does a good job of telling the reader that the skills she has learned as a massage therapist will suit her well as a physician assistant.

LONG-TERM GOALS

You may be asked to comment on you future plans in your essay, or in the interview. It may be unrealistic for an applicant to know exactly what she wants to do when finishing school. If you do have some definite plans, however, and you have something substantial to say, then by all mean mention it. But if you really have no definitive plans, then tell the committee that you are exploring several options and wish to keep an open mind at this time. Once you finish your clinical training, you may have a better idea.

PERSONAL PHILOSOPHY

This can be a very dangerous area, and while we all have our own convictions about certain topics, it is always best to keep on the conservative side. If you can speak intelligently and maturely about a topic that may give the reader some more insight into you as a person, then it may be permissible to speak on that subject. Avoid controversy at all costs, however. The last thing that you want to do is get involved in a controversy.

RE-APPLICANTS

You should definitely write a completely new essay this year. Be sure to mention how you have grown and what you have learned since last year. Also, send in fresh letters of reference along with your application. You must show that you have made some positive changes since your last application.

When you sit down to write your second essay, other issues and concerns may arise. We recommend that you think about the following:

1. Your initial thoughts after receiving your letter of rejection.
2. How you felt and reacted after the disappointment wore off.
3. Did you call the director of the program (post-interview) and ask why you were not accepted?
4. Your reaction to the director's comments and your subsequent behavior.
5. What have you done since speaking with the program director?
6. Have you made any progress since your last application?
7. Have you had any significant changes in grades or work experiences?
8. Why are you now a better candidate than last year?

Now it is time to re-write your essay from a re-applicant's point of view. Focus on the last question, *Why are you now a better candidate than last year?*

EVOLUTION OF AN ESSAY

The following essay is a first draft from a young woman applying to a PA school. After presenting the draft below, we will dissect it by paragraph and rewrite it so it is more effective.

When I was young; I vividly remember dressing up as a doctor for Halloween and dreaming of becoming one "When I grew up." At that early age, I viewed those in the health professions through rose colored glasses, as though I thought they could heroically heal people through an injection or a prescription. However, during a hospital internship my senior year, in high school, I realized that the OR is not always that miraculous center of recovery I had once envisioned. While observing a craniotomy, I watched a patient die on the operating table. I was shocked at the emotional distance the health care team showed, then realized death was something inevitable that health care

WHY ARE YOU NOW A BETTER CANDIDATE THAN LAST YEAR?

THE ESSAY

41

providers face everyday. The physicians, along with the rest of the health care team fulfilled their obligation; to try to cure the patient of a malignant brain tumor. It was then I learned that although modern medicine can prolong life, in the long run, it is death that wins because of the limitations of the human body. However, I decided that merely observing death impassively was beyond me, that I would wish to interact with the patients more intimately than the physician can.

After graduating high school, for two consecutive summers I interned for an orthopedic surgeon. Although I had seen PA's previously, the first time I really took note of one was outside the OR watching her comfort a patient just about to enter the OR. She was explaining exactly what was going to happen once the patient would enter the OR. I could tell that the patient deeply appreciated this extra attention he wouldn't have otherwise received. Later, while reviewing the patient's chart prior to his surgery, I struck up a conversation with an orthopedic PA. As we chatted outside the OR, she asked me whether I planned to go to medical school. Though I had always known I wanted to work in the health care field, I was not sure that I really wanted to become a physician. The aspect of diagnosing and treating patients was what I wanted to do. However, I did not want to spend the next ten to twelve years of my life in school, nor did I seek the confinement and lack of family time a doctor experiences. As my new friend described her profession, I could discern her enthusiasm for it and her caring personality, both of which struck a responsive chord within me. Until I met this PA, I was unaware of how my character and the traits requisite for being a PA coincide.

Every chance I received, I took advantage of my opportunities to investigate the functions of a PA. More and more I became interested in the PA's ability not only to make decisions autonomously but to work as a team with other physicians and nurses. I relish the notion of interacting directly with my patients and help select the optimal way to comfort and cure them. I was also struck by the PA program's versatility and flexibility, which allow me to change specialties if I desire. Being an independent thinker, as well as a people oriented individual, I have concluded that I am well suited not just for the medical field but for a lifetime career as a PA.

I look forward to this fall to furthering my experience with PA's, when I will be shadowing a PA in the ER of Austin's Brackenridge Hospital. I know that further acquaintance with this position will enhance my understanding of what, I hope, my life's career and help prepare me for its rigors and rewards. Nevertheless, I am already positive that I have found my true calling in life and eagerly anticipate working together with my PA colleagues assisting others to return to the sometimes rock-strewn road to good health. Because the operating room has always been my passion, I most likely will want to concentrate in that area, but as a highly receptive and open-minded person, I will be more than willing to change and focus in different spheres of health care if the occasion to do so arises.

In essence, my background in the medical field and witnessing many different procedures have convinced me that my lifetime dream can best come to reality through dedicating myself to a career as a PA.

L.L.

Paragraph #1. This young writer uses word pictures to try and make her essay more interesting. The problem is that her sentences are sometimes awkward and confuse the reader. She also, unintentionally, makes it sound as though the health care team is cold and uncaring instead of professional and objective. In addition, she uses abbreviations without first using the complete term. Finally, she speaks of death as being in competition with life; death is a part of life.

Paragraph #2. The opening sentence is awkward. She uses "PA's" instead of "PAs". She assumes that the patient would not have received the proper attention were it not for the PA. She uses the colloquial expression "chatted." She writes, ". . . nor did I seek the confinement and lack of family time a doctor experiences." In fact, one does not usually *seek* a negative. She also uses the improper tense at the beginning of this same sentence, ". . . I did not want to . . ." should be, ". . . I do not want to . . ."

Paragraph #3. In the first sentence the writer needs to explain when and where she took advantage of her opportunities to investigate the functions of PAs. She also has a big problem with tense. Since she is describing how she wants to become a PA, she should be writing either in the conditional tense, or in the future tense, stating, "I was also struck by the PA program's versatility and flexibility, which will allow me to change specialties if I desire."

Paragraph #4. This paragraph has numerous spelling and grammatical errors. She uses the colloquial term "rock strewn." She also becomes a little too subjective saying, ". . . as a highly receptive and open-minded person . . ."

Paragraph #5. Needs to be grammatically stronger without the participle "witnessing."

Here is the final version of the same essay.

When I was a child, I vividly remember dressing up as a doctor for Halloween. At that early age I viewed those in the health profession through rose-colored glasses, as if I thought they would heroically heal people through an injection or with a prescription. However, during a hospital internship in high school I realized that the operating room (OR) is not always the miraculous center of recovery I had envisaged. While observing a craniotomy I watched a patient die on the operating table. I was shocked that the health care team seemed to handle this with considerable objectivity and emotional distance, until I realized that death was an inevitability that health care providers face everyday. The physicians and other members of the health care team had fulfilled their obligation: to try to cure the patient of a malignant brain tumor. I learned that although modern medicine can prolong life, in the long run death is unavoidable because of the limitations of the human body. However, I decided that merely observing death impassively was beyond me and that I wanted to interact with patients more closely than a physician has the time to do.

After graduating from high school, I interned for an orthopedic surgeon for two consecutive summers. Although I had seen PAs previously, the first time I really took note of one was outside the OR watching her comfort a patient just about to undergo a surgical procedure. The PA explained exactly what was going to happen to him once he entered the room. I could tell that the patient deeply appreciated this extra attention as he began to smile and his face became more relaxed.

Later, while reviewing another patient's chart prior to her surgery, I began speaking with an orthopedic PA, Sherry. As we talked outside the holding area, she asked me whether I planned to go to medical school. Although I always knew I wanted to work in health care, I was not really sure that I wanted to become a physician. On the one hand I wanted the challenge of diagnosing and treating patients, but on the other hand I did not want to invest ten years of my life pursuing this goal. I also have plans of raising a family someday, and relish the idea of spending as much time as possible with them. As my new acquaintance described her profession, I could discern her enthusiasm for it and her caring personality, both of which struck a responsive chord in me. Until I met Sherry, I was unaware of how my character and the traits required for being a PA coincide.

Every chance I received after that meeting, I took advantage of my opportunities to investigate the functions of PAs working in various fields. More and more, I became interested in the PA's ability not only to make decisions autonomously, but also to work collaboratively with other members of the health care team. I look forward to being able to interact directly with my own patients and to, one day, be able to comfort them, and hopefully play a significant role in curing them, too. Being an independent thinker and working in a very versatile and flexible career are all very appealing to me.

This fall, I look forward to furthering my experience with PAs, when I will shadow a PA in the emergency room of Austin's Brackenridge Hospital. I am confident that further acquaintance with this position will enhance my understanding of what I hope will be my life's career and help prepare me for its rigors and rewards. Nevertheless, I am already positive that I have found my true calling in life, and eagerly anticipate working together with my PA colleagues assisting others to return on the sometimes difficult road to good health. Because the operating room is my passion, I will more than likely want to concentrate in surgery, but as a receptive and open-minded person, I will be willing to change and focus in different arenas of health care if the occasion to do so arises.

In essence, my background in the medical field and the fact that I have witnessed PAs working in various environments have convinced me that my lifetime dream can best come to fruition through dedicating myself to a career as a PA.

My other recommendation to this candidate was to provide examples of other skills, collaborative work experiences, and organizational duties or functions.

ESSAYS THAT WORKED

Sample #1

Attach to this application a typewritten narrative of not more than two pages, explaining where you learned of the PA profession, what factors or influences led you to this career choice, and how you expect to fulfill your goals as a physician associate.

For four years in the middle 1970s I was a Navy Corpsman, providing direct medical care to more than 400 marines, often in conditions of urgency and with little or no supervision. During this time I was exposed to the drama and trauma associated with medical care on a day-to-day basis. I learned how to work under conditions of limited or imperfect information and how to maintain composure under stress. Most importantly, I felt firsthand the profound satisfaction that comes from successfully delivering medical care.

After an Honorable Discharge from the Navy in 1979, I worked in the Yale-New Haven Hospital as an emergency room technician. During this time I had a chance to develop my skills as a team worker in a collaborative environment. This experience significantly broadened my view of disease and death, as the majority of our patients were not healthy young males as they tended to be in the military. I saw the direct effects of disease on infants, children, adolescents, adults, and elderly people of all ages, ethnic backgrounds, and socioeconomic conditions.

At Yale-New Haven, I worked closely with a physician associate. This was the first time I had ever been exposed to this career. His obvious technical expertise and medical knowledge were impressive. However, the profession was far less developed than it is today. I left the emergency room knowing that I wanted to pursue my career interests in health care, but unsure of which route to follow. I then decided to earn a four-year degree in Chemistry.

During my junior year in college, my career plans were changed drastically by the birth of my first child. Since I did not wish to continue to head a household as the proverbial "starving student," I decided upon graduating to rejoin the military, in this case the Air Force. This represented a degree of security to me for the time being.

For the past several years I have been an industrial salesperson. It has been quite rewarding from the point of view of allowing me to provide a good standard of living for myself and my family. However, it does not give me the deep satisfaction I receive from my hospital volunteer work. I have the feeling that the products I sell could be sold by anyone, but that service as a health professional is a genuine honor and calling.

So, what, at my age and professional level, is the best way to become a health professional? To attempt to go to medical school would be an enormous investment of time and money. I have considered nursing or acting as a nurse practitioner, but I am more interested in the technical and diagnostic aspects of medicine and the close partnership with a physician that being a physician associate can give.

In my deliberations over making this career choice, I have talked extensively with physicians, physician associates, and other health care professionals. I have taken further coursework and done well. One of the reasons that the profession of physician associate appeals to me as a long-term career choice is the opportunity to directly influence people in a positive way. Specifically, I am referring to the importance of continuing to emphasize in a strong but helpful way the basics of preventive medicine. In the past a relative and two close friends died from preventable diseases. This has dramatically shown me the responsibility a caregiver has in encouraging habits which prolong and improve the quality of life.

I have come to see and believe strongly in the concept that good medicine does not only come from bottles and boxes, but also from the heart and feelings of the caregiver. To be truly effective as a physician associate, I will have to excel in technical ability and medical knowledge, but also as a communicator. Very few people can, in the course of their work, help save or significantly prolong a life. As a physician associate, I will have the opportunity of taking a minute to talk about why stop smoking or go on a diet. This to me is a true measure of a career satisfaction.

One of the most valuable aspects of my experience has been the opportunity to work with and for outstanding individuals. These people are not only scientifically rigorous with information, but extremely humane in their dealings with others, both colleagues and patients. One such individual is a physician associate with whom I work at St. Raphael's Hospital. She is energetic, positive, personable, seems to always have a moment and a good word for everybody. Above all, she is a total professional and earns by her daily efforts the respect of those she works with.

The Physician Associate Program is an ideal way to realize career ambitions in health care. Physician associates have the chance to act at a significant level of intervention with patients without needing to invest the years and years of training that becoming a physician would require.

If given the opportunity, I plan to use my physician associate training to return to the Emergency Room in a newly enhanced role. This, to me, is where so much of the opportunity exists to practice the skills I have and will develop. I enjoy the direct contact with people, the fast-changing environment, and most of all the chance to directly work with and help people who are in serious need. With the AIDS epidemic, the prevalence of teen violence, and the enormous substance abuse problems today, I am sure that there will be more need than ever for skilled, competent individuals to assist in this critical area.

A.J.R.

Sample #2
Tell the committee what factors led you to choose a career as a physician assistant, and how you have prepared yourself for this role.

My decision to seek a career in medicine was influenced by several personal and work-based experiences. However, it was my grandfather, a very important person in my life, who played a significant role in finalizing my career choice. Shortly after my thirteenth birthday, he was hospitalized with a heart attack. He subsequently underwent heart surgery and suffered a stroke in the immediate post-operative period. I felt overwhelmed by the fact that no one seemed to be able to do anything to help him. One day while I sat at his bedside I realized that I wanted to get involved in medicine, and I promised him that I would work hard to be able to help others get well. The next week he died, and I became more determined than ever to make a difference by caring for others.

Over the last several years, my interest in becoming a physician assistant has been strengthened by my extracurricular and work activities. While in high school I worked as a unit clerk, part-time, on a busy surgical floor. It was here that I was briefly introduced to the work of PAs. My duties consisted of answering the phone, ordering lab tests, and, at times, interacting with the patients. As a result of this exposure, I became familiar with medical terminology, learned about the health care "team" concept, and played a significant role in recruiting volunteers to our floor to spend time with our patients. During the summer of 1990, I received my first "hands-on" experience and my first direct contact with PAs. I worked as a technician in the emergency room alongside nurses, doctors, technicians, and PAs. I collected and measured vital signs, obtained short medical histories, assisted in trauma cases, and sometimes just held a patient's hand to comfort her. It was here that I learned that the practice of medicine is as much about good care-giving as it is about the appropriate drug therapy.

In 1992, while studying chemistry at Southern University, I participated in numerous extracurricular activities, thus enhancing my leadership and interpersonal skills. These activities provided situations in which I was allowed to exercise my capabilities as president, vice-president, treasurer, and secretary. For instance, in my role as president of the Spanish Club, I initiated activities such as a winter coat drive for inner city Hispanic children, and worked with a team of community leaders and students to achieve our goal of collecting over 1000 coats.

I have also been involved in other activities which have given me the opportunity to help those who are socio-economically disadvantaged and unable to care for themselves. This volunteer work ranged from working at the Saint Ann's soup kitchen and reading to the blind, to holding and feeding "crack babies" in the Newborn Intensive Care Unit at Michener Hospital. As a result of these experiences, I learned to reach out to others and help make a positive change in their lives. I also made quite a few new friends along the way. At Michener Hospital, I also worked on the crisis hot-line where my responsibilities were to be an attentive, confident listener and to provide the caller with reference information pertinent to the inquiry. Through this experience I have gained confidence in dealing with crisis situations.

During my senior year at Southern, I was employed by the local Veteran's Hospital as a cardiac rehabilitation aide. I worked very closely with patients either recovering from bypass surgery or from heart attacks. I walked with patients, counseled them on proper nutrition, and helped develop an exercise regimen for the "Take Heart" program. This experience improved my ability to listen to patients and to teach them at the same time.

Presently, I am a volunteer with the Orange County Fire Department. I work as an EMT. This experience is teaching me how to work under extreme conditions of stress.

My desire to become a physician assistant is sincere and founded on a working knowledge of the role of PAs. I am committed to doing whatever is necessary to achieve my goal.

D.K.

Sample #3

This applicant was accepted to every program that she applied to: Duke, Yale, Northeastern, and George Washington. She has a rich cultural and ethnic history, and she uses her experiences very effectively.

The majority of my extracurricular activities falls under the following categories:

A) Music

I began to take flute lessons in 1974 at the age of seven and at thirteen also began violin lessons. I have become quite accomplished on both instruments and have played in various musical ensembles. Presently I play first-flute in the Stratford, Connecticut Community Band, of which I am the youngest member, and first-flute in the Fairfield University Flute Choir, which I helped organize in 1986. From 1981 to 1983, I played first violin in the Bridgeport, Connecticut Youth Symphony, and the Sherwood Orchestra. Other ensembles include the Fairfield University Chamber Orchestra and groups annually assembled by my music teachers to regularly perform for residents of convalescent homes. Over the years I have also played in local bands and done solo performances at various private parties and organizational functions.

B) Ethnic Activities

My home life is quite unique in that my parents are immigrants from Czecho-Slovakia and as a result I am able to speak, read, and write the Slovak language fluently. I greatly value my Slovak heritage and culture, and thus a great deal of my time is spent on ethnic activities.

From 1986 to 1987, I served as the General Chairman of the centennial celebration of the St. John Nepomucene Society, the oldest Slovak fraternal society in New England. My leadership abilities were strengthened by this event for, having been given a free hand by the society officers, I directed all arrangements and preparations. This year-long activity culminated in a successful weekend program highlighted by religious services and a banquet attended by over 360 people.

In August 1988, I was selected to be a delegate to the 32nd National Convention of the "First Slovak Wreath of the Free Eagle," a national Slovak-American fraternal society which was organized in 1986. At the convention I was appointed to serve on the by-laws committee and as assistant secretary of the convention. I was also honored by being elected to the office of Supreme Youth Director. Not only was I the youngest member in attendance at the convention, but also the youngest, in the ninety-two year history of the organization, to be elected to the Board of Directors.

To conserve and perpetuate our Slovak culture and traditions, the Slovak societies also sponsor weekly radio programs which I help produce. At WWPT, Westport, Connecticut, I help produce and coordinate the "Slovak Alliance Program," which presents traditional folk songs from Slovakia. At WSHU, Fairfield, Connecticut, I help produce and coordinate "Music from Slovakia," which presents both classical and traditional music written or performed by Slovak composers and ensembles.

C) Work Experience

To help finance my education I work throughout the year. From September 1984 to May 1987, I was a counter worker at a dry-cleaning establishment, averaging thirty-five hours per week during the school year and fifty hours per week during the summer months. A most enjoyable aspect of this job was the constant contact I had with the public. The interaction with various people certainly sharpened my social skills.

From June 1987 to present, I have worked for a dermatologist and average twenty-five hours per week. As a medical assistant at the physician's office, I have gotten hands-on experience and insight into how a physician works in a private practice and how a medical office is run. My duties range from reception to assisting the doctor or nurse.

As a receptionist, I log in patients and make them feel comfortable and answer questions regarding medications, services, and surgeries. The clerical aspect includes typing referral letters and reports, billing, and handling health insurance claims. I often assist the doctor with minor surgery, which also includes preparing specimens for the Pathology lab and charting. Most interesting has been my observation of and assistance with hair transplantation surgery, microscopic work, and phlebotomy necessary for the "Fibrel" injections used in scar and wrinkle treatment. At the office I also make up solutions of Minoxidil used in the treatment of hair loss, monitor the blood pressure of Minoxidil patients, and make up a moisturizing cream with Tretinoin (Retin A) used to prevent skin wrinkles and acne.

In addition, I am presently a teaching assistant for the Freshman Biology lab at Fairfield University, a volunteer therapist's assistant for a program for handicapped children, and will soon be certified to perform cardiopulmonary resuscitation (CPR). My experiences in the health care field are quite varied and have not only expanded my medical knowledge but have also provided me with valuable practical experience.

D) Miscellaneous

My other community activities include working as a volunteer at the Easter Seals Rehabilitation Center, Bridgeport, Connecticut, where I work with young children suffering mental and physical handicaps. I also volunteer my time at the Merton House soup kitchen, Bridgeport, Connecticut, which provides food and clothing for the poor and homeless.

E) Why I Want to Pursue a Career in Medicine

Sometimes a person experiences one significant event which changes her life and outlook. For me it occurred in 1978 when my father suffered a severe skull fracture due to a fall from a ladder. He remained in a coma for five days but, luckily, he completely recovered from his injuries. This close encounter with death left me with a greater appreciation of, and respect for, life. Most importantly, however, this experience gave me an incentive. I am forever indebted to God and to the physicians for caring for my father's life, and my career choice is my way of repaying this debt. I am willing to make many more sacrifices in order to achieve my goal, and if I can help others just as my father was helped, and if I can inspire someone just as I was inspired, I know all of my work and sacrifice will not be in vain. This calling comes from deep within me, and I am confident that I can and will achieve my goal.

L.H.

Sample #4

The focus of this candidate's essay is on making a career change. She is also an "older" applicant.

My first exposure to the Physician Associate profession was in 1983 when I was treated for a minor medical problem by a PA at CHCP. I asked the universal question of "What is a PA?" and spoke with the PA briefly about his work. Since then I have had regular contact with PAs through my health insurance providers. Once I seriously considered the PA profession for myself, I read professional journals, the Physician Assistant Journal and the Journal of the American Academy of Physician Assistants, and talked with PAs to learn more about the profession.

I am currently looking to make a change in my career. The last couple of years have been a time for reflection and change, with a focus on reviewing my career objectives. I have come to the conclusion that I want to be involved in a career that:

▶ Has a bright future
▶ Is directly involved with people
▶ Is in the medical arena
▶ Meets my need for continuing education and opportunity for change
▶ Will utilize my past life/work experiences and skills

The Physician Associate profession meets all of these criteria.

There is no question as to the viability of the profession. Certainly, the creation of a national health care system which demands affordable health care will only increase that need. Indicators predict that the PA profession will be growing for the next decade and beyond. I still have another 20–25 years of work ahead of me and want my next profession to be one that will offer a lot of opportunity.

My need to be involved with people has been life-long. I have been able to meet this need through volunteer experiences as well as through the evolution of my career. In my first position as a Horticulture Manager, I worked directly with individuals who have differing needs, planning and providing vocational rehabilitation programs. I met with their families and, at times, found myself in situations which were emotional and challenging. As Personnel Director, I have worked with staff, applicants, and volunteers in areas of hiring, firing, terminal illness, addictions, work-related injuries, and performance issues.

Within this area I have had to make tough decisions without letting my personal bias interfere. With these previous experiences, I have developed strong interpersonal skills which will be a substantial asset to me as a PA.

I now find that I want to become involved with people at a more critical level, focusing on their good health and wellness. My original career interests took me in many different directions. I was very interested in physical therapy and the human sciences but also had a strong attraction to horticulture and the plant sciences. My decision to enter the field of horticulture therapy came when I learned that I could combine my two areas of interest. After 5 years of providing hands-on services in a vocational rehabilitation environment, I felt the need to become part of the administrative team and entered graduate school to study organization and management. Now that I have been in administration for 8 years, I find that my interests are pulling me into the medical field again.

As my life progresses, I have observed in myself the need for a profession that offers a diverse array of opportunities. In addition to the diversity of a PA's career options, I find it revitalizing to be in a profession that requires continuing education. The prospect of a career with broad possibilities and education expansion is both attractive and motivational.

Changing my career will only make sense if I can utilize my past work experiences and skills. It is in this area that I feel I will be able to give the most back to the PA profession. In my 15 years with SARAH, I have developed and implemented both the horticulture and personnel departments from infancy. I now am in the process of implementing yet another new department for SARAH, quality evaluation, for which I will be the Director. As the PA profession continues to flourish, there will be a need for people with an administrative and management background such as mine to create and administer the growing number of programs and services PAs will be providing.

I consider returning to school as an "older student" a very exciting opportunity. The time I spent at Antioch New England Graduate School was one of the most stimulating periods of my life, thus far. The experience of working 40 hours per week at SARAH and going to school nights in Hartford and weekends in Keene, New Hampshire, lifted me to a level of energy and motivation that was both stimulating and rewarding. I believe that I will be very successful entering _____ PA program, with its intensive and rigorous curriculum, given my success at Antioch. I look forward to the challenge with excitement and confidence.

At this point in my life, a career move requires much thought and consideration. After reassessing my career options, I feel that this is the time to make a move. The Physician Associate profession will bring me back to my original interest in medicine and meet all of my career objectives. By combining my successful educational and work history with my original desire and aptitude in the physical sciences, I am confident that you will find me to be an excellent candidate for your program.

I look forward to having the opportunity to meet with you in an interview for student selection to further discuss my interest in _____ Physician Associate program.

T.S.

What follows are several annotated essay examples, and a selection of paragraphs from essays. These examples may further help you when constructing your own narrative.

Annotated Essay 1

Charles Boelter

The first time I can recall meeting a Physician Assistant was in the emergency room of Martin Army Community Hospital, on Fort Benning, Georgia. I was a private, going through basic infantry training, and happened to be clumsy enough to fall from the top of the forty-foot rope climb on the obstacle course. I knew he was an officer, but he obviously was neither a doctor nor a nurse. He pulled a large piece of wood from under my thumbnail and sent me for some x-rays. He determined that I was not mortally wounded, and released me to my unit.

I managed to survive basic training, and eventually I wound up as a paratrooper in the Eighty-Second Airborne Division. Throughout the course of my enlistment, I was able to spend a considerable amount of time with our battalion PA. I learned what he did and what options his profession provided him. When the time came for me to leave active duty, I was beginning to think about the Physician Assistant profession as a career path.

I have wanted a career in medicine for as long as I can remember. I am sure this is because of my father, and the stories I have heard about him. He learned the intricacies of medicine in school, but he was born with the innate ability to care for, and about, people.

We lived in a small town, amidst a million acres of corn, in rural Illinois. My father practiced from a small office that was actually our converted garage. From this office he took care of the people in our town, on the surrounding farms, and those in the nearby communities. Less than one month after my brother was born, our father left on a house call from which he never returned. He died that night, leaving his sons a legacy of caring and competency that I hear about to this day. My brother never felt the calling of the medical profession as strongly as I have, so he offered encouragement and support to help me achieve my goals. His encouragement stopped when he was killed

OPENING PARAGRAPH USES A SCENARIO WITH IMMEDIACY TO GAIN THE ATTENTION OF THE READER

OUTLINES INTEREST IN THE PA PROFESSION

IDENTIFIES A MORE DEEPLY FELT MOTIVATION

STRONG PERSONAL AND EMOTIONAL EXPERIENCES ARE STATED WITH RESTRAINT shortly after I left the military. His death left me as the only one to follow in my father's footsteps.

My life has prepared me for a career as a Physician Assistant in many ways. I believe that, like my father, I have an innate ability to care about people and what happens to them. I want to help make positive changes in their lives much as my father did. Being a leader taught me to be responsible for myself, and for my subordinates. I learned not only how to make decisions, but also to recognize the consequences those decisions might have. My work as a medical assistant has given me a better understanding of how the medical team works together to satisfy patient needs. It has exposed me to clinical decision making and the complexities of modern medicine. I have seen first hand the role Physician Assistants fulfill in the medical community, and how they fit into the team approach to care, by shadowing them in various settings. I believe I have been given the character and the ability to become a competent Physician Assistant.

My strongest desire in life is to experience the joys and rigors of a profession in medicine much as my father did. I have the ability and desire to help people, but I need the tools to do this. Becoming a Physician Assistant will give me the tools I need to take the next step in my career. This is the path I am on, and it is where I can offer the most for those who need help.

Annotated Essay #2

Yvonne Gonzalez

My interest in becoming a Physician Associate (PA) is rooted in the desire to provide quality health care to the underprivileged—whose health care needs I have perceived to be acute in the course of my volunteer work. As a Social Justice Coordinator for my parish, I organized volunteer efforts at a number of facilities: pediatric clinics and orphanages in Baja, California, the L.A. Mission and the Catholic Worker (a soup kitchen and free clinic in L.A.). I also represented the parish in a 10-day, 250-mile walk-athon from Santa Barbara to Tijuana to raise money for a child welfare agency. I have never felt so much satisfaction in my career achievements as compared to the gratification I derive from working with the underprivileged. Their acute health care needs prompted my desire to become involved in a professional capacity. I felt frustrated, however, because I did not want to become a physician and just could not see myself in any of the allied health careers. It was not until I learned of the Physician Associate profession that I realized I could fulfill my dream of working in public health at a significant level of medical intervention without having to train for 8 or more years.

I first learned of Physician Associates when my father had a double bypass in 1994 and his post-operative care was managed by his cardiologist's staff PA, Helen. When she explained her role to me, I was impressed with the scope of her responsibilities and sensed that this might be the opportunity I had been seeking. Not long after I met Helen, I began shadowing Ted Braunstein, a PA in the Emergency Department of Mount Sinai Medical Center. I was impressed by his clinical knowledge, compassion, and aptitude for patient education. I was also surprised to see the degree of autonomy given Ted by the attending physicians. We worked out a pact: Ted would answer all of my questions and I would help him obtain histories and physicals on Spanish-speaking patients. I soon found myself assisting the patient representatives when they were short-handed. It wasn't long before I was gloving up to help steady patients as Ted performed suturing of lumbar punctures. Next, the technicians taught me how to draw blood, insert Foley catheters, and take vital measurements. Even after over 1500 hours, I am still amazed at the fascinating array of patients and clinical challenges every shift offers.

EVIDENCE OF SELF-REFLECTION AND UNDERSTANDING OF HIS OWN SKILLS AND ABILITIES

RE-CAPS HIS REASONS FOR WANTING TO BECOME A PA IN A SUCCINCT CONCLUSION

CLEAR OPENING SENTENCE WHICH PAVES THE WAY FOR FURTHER SUPPORTING EVIDENCE

STRONG HISTORY OF VOLUNTEER WORK AND UNDERSTANDING OF SOCIAL JUSTICE ISSUES

FOCUSES ON HER INITIAL INTEREST IN THE PROFESSION AND THEN BUILDS ON HOW IT DEVELOPED FURTHER INTO A LIFELONG GOAL

USE OF HER OWN BACKGROUND AND LANGUAGE SKILLS TO IMPROVE PATIENT ACCESS TO CARE. SPECIFICALLY LISTS THE SKILLS SHE ACQUIRED

CLEAR VISION OF WHERE SHE
WANTS TO BE IN THE FUTURE

USES A NEW SLANT ON HER
SKILLS TO CONSOLIDATE THE
ESSAY

STRONG, UNUSUAL BEGINNING
PARAGRAPH LINKED TO THE
DESIRE TO STUDY MEDICINE

EFFECT OF A PERSONAL
EXPERIENCE WHICH BECOMES A
TURNING POINT

ANOTHER KEY TURNING POINT

If given the opportunity, I plan to use my PA training to work in public health. Ideally, I would like to divide my time between an urban tertiary care facility and a rural clinic. Working in such diverse settings will, I feel, provide me with a strong clinical foundation and the opportunity for continuing education that will benefit both patient populations. Serving those in serious need will fulfill a lifelong goal and doing so in a PA capacity will allow me to utilize the analytical, communication, and time-management skills I have acquired in my career thus far. My decision to become a PA is based on a working knowledge of the role of the PA, and I am committed to making the necessary sacrifices to achieve this goal.

Annotated Essay #3

Norman deDios

I have always been fascinated by the mysteries of nature. While my boyhood friends admired Batman, I idolized Jacques Cousteau. To me, he represented man's unrelenting desire to explore the unknown, while demonstrating a deep respect for the natural order of living things. As a child, I consumed countless books on science and spent hours watching documentaries trying to understand the "hows" and "whys" of life. I even went so far as to set up my own "pet shop" in our basement which eventually contained one hundred tropical fish, ranging from a feisty red-eyed South American Manguenese to a two-foot-long Silver Arrowana. It is this innate curiosity that has evolved into and become the foundation of my desire to study medicine.

My interest in the natural world took a personal and painful turn when I was awakened to the reality of human beings suffering during my sophomore year at Providence College. At that time, my father suffered a major heart attack, for which he required quadruple bypass surgery and a four-week stay in hospital. It was frightening to see the man who always seemed invincible to me lying in a hospital attached to so many machines. My father's illness forced me to redefine my role in the family and I suddenly found myself at its head. During this time I traveled regularly from Providence to New Haven to look after my father and provide support to my mother and siblings. Unfortunately, this sudden shift of responsibility and unfamiliar stress was reflected in my poor grades. The fragility of life and the importance of family became clear to me, and I realized that this difficult period would serve as a transition point toward a new level of maturity, a maturity that strengthened my ability to persevere and heightened my feelings of compassion and concern for others.

My work experience in health care began with a summer job as a Laboratory Assistant in the Blood Chemistry Laboratory of the Hospital of St. Raphael. My responsibilities included keeping records of blood specimens as well as interacting directly with physicians and other members of the hospital staff. The following summer, I was employed as an Operating Room Aide in the Ambulatory Surgery Unit of Yale-New Haven Hospital, where contact with patients on a personal level was a new and rewarding experience. My job gave me the opportunity to interact with patients before their surgery and also upon their discharge. It was extremely gratifying to know that the support I offered these patients was not only reassuring but also greatly appreciated. I have always felt a tremendous amount of self-reward knowing that I made a difference in a person's life, simply by showing them I cared. It was this personal time with patients that proved to be the most satisfying aspect of my job at Yale-New Haven and further motivated me to pursue a career in the health sciences.

After graduating from college, I accepted a position as a research assistant at Yale University School of Medicine, Department of OB/GYN. Working closely with Drs. Aydin Arici and Ibrahim Sozen on their Leiomyoma research, I aided in the completion of their study on the effects of growth factor-B1 on myometrial tumors. Our work will be published in the near future. After completing my work with Drs. Arici and Sozen, I was given the opportunity to work with David Keefe, also of Yale's OB/GYN Department. I thoroughly enjoyed my time with Dr. Keefe due to his confidence in me to work unsupervised and because of the relationship we formed as I occasionally accompanied him throughout his busy day seeing patients. It was with Dr. Keefe that I gained an understanding and appreciation for the intimacy and trust patients have in their health care provider.

WORK OUTCOMES CLEARLY STATED

After leaving Yale, I continued to work in the field of research as a Laboratory Assistant in the Department of Molecular Genetics at New York Medical College. This laboratory was involved in the identification of the gene that caused ataxia telangiectasia, a nueromolecular disease that strikes young children. My responsibilities included cataloging daily blood specimens and isolating DNA for gene identification. Although my role was a small one, it was gratifying to know that my work may aid others in eventually finding a cure for this disease.

LEARNING FROM OTHERS

While I enjoyed my research, I missed the personal contact I had with patients. This led me to spend this past summer shadowing physician assistants in the Cardiothoracic Unit at The Hospital of St. Raphael, which rekindled my interest in clinical medicine. This experience has clarified my image of a physician assistant's role in health care, as well as given me a better understanding of where I hope to be in this field. My interest in patient care has been further enhanced by my current volunteer work with Yale-New Haven Hospital Elderlife Program. This position allows me to work one-on-one with geriatric patients and has given me hands-on experience in the health care field. I also feel that volunteer work continues to develop techniques for communicating and interacting with patients that I will use in my career as a physician assistant.

REMINDS THE READER OF ONE OF THE KEY FACTORS FOR HIM IN WISHING TO BECOME A PA

Another area in which I have been able to refine my interpersonal skills has been through my involvement in music. At ten years of age, my friends and I formed a band in which we all continue to perform. As the keyboard player, a vocalist, and a guitarist, I realize that the ability to share and relate ideas is essential to being a successful and unified group. Through music, I have learned the value of patience, cooperation, and understanding, and strive to utilize these qualities in everyday life.

GOOD EXAMPLE OF TRANSFERABLE SKILLS—THOSE SKILLS ACQUIRED IN ANOTHER AREA WHICH WILL BE USEFUL IN THE PA PROFESSION

I believe that the adversities I have faced have helped me to mature, and I regard them as growing stages in my life. These events have affected me because I genuinely do care about others, and they have shown me how committed and determined I am. I sincerely believe that I now possess the qualities to become a responsible, compassionate, and caring physician assistant. Therefore, I refuse to let these obstacles discourage me and to this day I am continuing my education as well as my involvement in health care. I look forward to using my newly found reservoir of strength toward a lifelong career in medicine. My experiences in health care, and my interactions with physician assistants have only strengthened my resolve. I know that as time passes, I can use my experiences, both positive and negative, to become a truly competent physician assistant.

CLEAR REITERATION OF WHAT HE HAS SAID BEFORE WITH A SLIGHTLY DIFFERENT FOCUS.

EXAMPLES OF ESSAY EXTRACTS

OPENING PARAGRAPHS

Imagine waking every day of the year at four o'clock in the morning to care for one hundred head of dairy cattle. This is what my wife Carla and I have done for the past seventeen years. . . .

Bradford Phillips

During the past years, I have worked with or shadowed four exceptional Physician Assistants who have given me valuable insight to the PA profession. As I worked with these health care providers, I analyzed their skills and qualities and inventoried their commonalities. Besides maintaining a high level of technical proficiency, each of them is a superior team leader, outstanding communicator, and creative problem solver. My formal education in psychology and my personal experiences have provided me with an opportunity to develop those three vital qualities.

Amy Fritsch

The inextricable relationship between health and mental health has intrigued me for over fourteen years. As a teenager, I watched programs on public television about the etiology of psychotic disorders. After graduating from high school, I decided to follow my natural interests into the world of health care, earning degrees in mental health, psychology, and social work. With each educational milestone I have gained knowledge and experience that has enhanced my understanding of how to help others in need.

Barbara Ann Slusher

Examples of a Learning Experience That Had an Impact on an Individual in Shaping His/Her Aspirations

A few years ago I had occasion to reassess where I was in life, and where I had expected to be at this point. I found that the two did not match, and in fact bore little resemblance to each other. It was time to make up my own mind about where and how I spend the rest of my life. The task then became one of determining what track I wanted my life to be on, and how I was going to get there. One of the steps in my search led me to volunteer on the Neurology/Neurosurgery Nursing Unit at the George Washington University Medical Center—the first volunteer they had ever had. I quickly realized I not only felt very comfortable in the medical environment, but had also found a piece of what was missing in my life. Volunteering was good, and quite rewarding, but not nearly enough. I needed to be working in a medical field full time, and be in a position to provide patient care.

Jean Caldwell

The most poignant experience of my career that truly sparked my interest in medicine was my experience as a counselor in a methadone maintenance program. Our treatment team noticed marked improvements in the physical and mental health of our clients after only a short period of methadone treatment. It seemed that heroin addiction was a disease easily treated with methadone. What was confusing, however, was the high rate of relapse for clients who had successfully detoxified from the methadone after years of stable treatment.

Why did clients with such a positive prognosis and years of treatment relapse? We found that many factors influenced a client's ability to remain abstinent from drugs: lifestyle, HIV status, family history, socioeconomic status, et cetera. The relation between these factors was very complex. We could not treat just the physical aspect of the addiction and hope to be successful. For me, this learning experience underlined the fact that disease is not one dimensional. The best treatment approach is one that encompasses the physical, mental, and socio-emotional aspects of the individual in their environment.

Barbara Ann Slusher

. . . Although I had various responsibilities at the clinic, what stands out most in my mind was the time I spent listening, counseling, and teaching patients, and the tremendous satisfaction that came from this interaction. One woman

I remember came in to see the internist. After a thorough exam and some laboratory tests, the doctor told her that she had diabetes and was going to have to begin insulin therapy. I translated since she spoke only Spanish and could not understand what the doctor was saying. She only asked a few questions and seemed very hesitant and frightened about her future. We reassured her that she was in good hands and we would all be there to support her with the steps she needed to take. A few days later she returned to learn about diabetes management and insulin injections, and again I translated for her. For both the nurse and me it was challenging because she was apprehensive and doubtful that she was going to be able to manage everything by herself. We reassured her that although it was going to be difficult in the beginning, she could do it. We sat with her as she practiced the various tasks, from testing her blood sugar level and giving herself an injection to documenting everything in her journal. After about an hour she was ready to go home, feeling more comfortable with her daily routine. As she left, she took my hand and thanked me for my patience and support, telling me what a good person I was. It seemed strange that she would thank me for this, but her gratitude showed me how important it is to take time to listen, counsel, and support patients.

Katherine Coleman

EXAMPLE OF A STRONG CONCLUSION

These volunteer experiences have crystallized the challenges, rewards, and frustrations of being a health care provider, as well as the shortcomings of health care in the United States. These diverse environments have augmented my studies in public health, and have provided me with concrete examples of how individuals can benefit from caring, sensitive providers, and how communities suffer when adequate health care services are not available or affordable. As a Physician Assistant I will be poised to deliver health care services to under-served urban populations, and I will demonstrate compassion and sensitivity. Furthermore, the intensive, rigorous PA program at . . . will enable me to execute this career change effectively and efficiently.

Lynn R. Fryer

WORK HISTORY SHEET

Employer name: _____

Address: _____

Phone #: _____

Full time:_____   Part time: _____

Dates of employment: From:_____   To:_____

Job Title:_____

Job Description: (3 sentences or less)_____

_____

_____

_____

_____

Skills utilized: _____

Awards/citations: _____

Other information: _____

MEDICAL EXPERIENCE SHEET

Employer name: _____

Address:_____

Phone #: _____

months worked: Full time:_____   Part time: _____

Dates of employment:_____

Job title: (3 sentences or less) _____

_____

_____

_____

_____

Skills utilized (e.g. phlebotomy, vital signs, physical exams):_____

_____

Awards/citations:_____

Describe your most memorable patient (3 sentences or less):

_____

_____

_____

_____

Other information: _____

HIGH SCHOOL INFORMATION SHEET

High school attended: _____

Address:_____

Dates attended: From _____ To: _____

Major course of study: _____

GPA: _____

Team sports: _____

Clubs: _____

Awards/honors: _____

Volunteer work: _____

Other: _____

COLLEGE INFORMATION SHEET

College/University attended:_____

Address:_____

Dates attended: From _____ To: _____

Major:_____

Highest degree obtained: _____

GPA: _____

Team sports: _____

Clubs: _____

Volunteer work: _____

Awards/honors: _____

Did you work?:   yes___   no___

List one person whom you can contact for a good reference: ____

_____

Scholarships: _____

Other: _____

VOLUNTEER WORK

Volunteer description: _____

Why this position?: _____

Address:_____

Point of contact: _____

How long?:_____

Awards/letters of appreciation: _____

Most memorable patient/experience: _____

List one person who will write a good reference for you: _____

_____

MILITARY SERVICE

Branch of service: _____

Dates of service:_____

Type of discharge (honorable, general, etc.): _____

Where stationed?: _____

Job title (M.O.S.):_____

Supervisor: _____

Awards/ribbons/medals: _____

Special schools/training: _____

Did you attend college in the military?:_____

What did you learn from the experience? (teamwork, discipline, etc.): _____

_____

FOREIGN LANGUAGE

Do you speak a foreign language?:_____

What language: _____

How did you learn the language?:_____

TRAVEL

Where to?: _____

When?: _____

What did you learn from the experience?: _____

_____

_____

SPECIAL AWARDS/CITATIONS

Award type: _____

Why received?: _____

When received?: _____

Given by: _____

What did you do to get it?: _____

The Interview
(Part One)

7

The next three chapters will focus on various aspects of the interview process. In this chapter (Part One) I focus on some of the necessary skills you must have or acquire to be a strong applicant. I also provide you with some insight relative to the interview process as seen through the eyes of an applicant who failed her first try, but was accepted the next year. In the next chapter, I give you an overview of the interview process and teach you how to prepare for it. I explain the different types of interviews (group, individual, and student) and introduce you to the scoring process. In the third chapter, I provide you with actual interview questions and answers so you can maximize your preparation for the big day.

INTRODUCTION

Every PA school receives hundreds of applications each year. Once your application is received, the registrar will check it for completeness and forward it on for review by the admissions committee. Two committee members will review your application, give you a numerical score, and make a decision as to your interview status. Approximately 100 applicants are invited to interview. There is only one program that I am aware of that does not interview; Cuyahoga Community College in Ohio uses an extensive questionnaire to screen and evaluate candidates for acceptance.

It is important to mention that an applicant should not be too aggressive in seeking an interview. Never call a PA program and request or demand an interview. The decision to interview a candidate rests solely with the admissions committee. Students who call to request or demand an interview are not looked upon favorably. In fact, each time you contact the program and speak with an administrator, a note is usually placed in your file as to the reason for the call. You certainly do not want any unfavorable information placed in your file that will compromise your chances for acceptance. You may call the program to inquire if you will be invited for an interview, but only after the application deadline has passed by several weeks.

HOW IMPORTANT IS THE INTERVIEW?

At this point in the application process, you should realize that the interview is all that counts. Everything else—your education, work experience,

NEVER CALL A PA PROGRAM AND REQUEST OR DEMAND AN INTERVIEW.

essay, test scores—is simply support for this crucial meeting. Remember that statistics are cold and cerebral. Just because you have a 4.0 grade point average and you scored 1400 on your SATs does not mean that you are automatically going to be accepted into PA school.

At this point in the process, the admissions committee wants to learn more about you as a person. Are you likeable? Are you compassionate? Do you fully understand the role of the PA? Are you mature? Can you handle stress? Can the interviewer visualize you as a colleague? Are you overconfident? Are you trustworthy? Are you energetic? Would the interviewer want you taking care of him or her as a patient? Are you an effective communicator? The interview is your chance to sell yourself to the committee. Your grades, SAT scores, and essay were already good enough to get you this far. It is now time to concentrate on making an emotional connection with all of the committee members.

HIGH-IMPACT COMMUNICATION

If you are going to win a position in next year's class, you need to develop certain skills and behaviors that will enhance your position. The first of these behaviors is charisma. Funk and Wagnall's dictionary defines charisma as **extraordinary personal power or charm.** To some, charisma comes naturally, but more often than not it must be learned. Charisma is the result of a series of behaviors through which someone has a powerful and positive impact on others. This is exactly what we want to accomplish at the interview; use charisma to build the bridge to credibility and trust.

I interviewed many applicants who simply could not make a connection at the interview. These applicants could not move beyond facts, figures, and jargon to make that connection. In contrast, the applicants who scored the highest at the interview knew how to communicate effectively and persuasively, and above all, were absolutely believable. They understood how to project openness, enthusiasm, and energy. The ability to communicate effectively is the single most important skill you need to succeed as a PA.

Communication is a contact sport. As mentioned already, looking good on paper will only get you so far. If you are unable to make an emotional connection with your audience, you're likely to be rejected. I witnessed this phenomenon over and over again when I interviewed applicants. Although some candidates were only average on paper, they made such an emotional impact at the interview that I scored them higher than I had anticipated based on their application alone.

CREATING EMOTIONAL IMPACT

You must learn to sell yourself to create emotional impact. While preparing for one of my seminars, I received an e-mail from a person on the staff of a PA program in the southern United States. He wanted to "join the team" and help me out with my upcoming seminar in his location. I wrote back thanking him for his interest, but told him that I was not looking to hire anyone at this point. A week later, I received a telephone call from another PA wanting to come aboard and help me out with my seminars. This person, Chris, told me that he had seven years' experience on one of the local PA programs' admissions committees. He sold me on the idea that he would truly be an asset to my seminar program. He understood the power of the *liv-*

THE ABILITY TO COMMUNICATE
EFFECTIVELY IS THE SINGLE
MOST IMPORTANT SKILL YOU
NEED TO SUCCEED AS A PA.

COMMUNICATION IS A CONTACT
SPORT.

ing resume versus sending an e-mail. Chris understood that he was selling himself and I offered him a position.

What are you selling? Have you thought about it? Some people get uncomfortable when I mention the word "selling." They fail to realize that we all sell ourselves every day. We sell our ideas to our employers. We sell our crucial decisions to our spouses and loved ones. You will have to sell yourself to the admissions committee and give them a reason to invite you into the next class of PA school students.

The Secret

If I can get you to buy into the fact that we are all selling something, then you must also understand this crucial point: **The admissions committee selects candidates based on emotion and justifies its decision with facts.** If you can grasp this "secret" you will realize why I emphasize the fact that you cannot rely on your paper application to get you accepted; rather you must make an emotional connection with the committee.

After a candidate walks out of the interview room, the committee doesn't sit down with a legal pad and draw a line down the center separating your strengths and weaknesses. Your score, and the ultimate decision of whether to accept you into the program, is mainly influenced by emotional factors versus rational factors alone. If the committee liked you at an emotional level, it will justify giving you a higher score by commenting favorably on your grade point average, SAT scores, medical experience, or whatever will work to support this emotionally based decision. If the committee doesn't like you at an emotional level, you can have a 4.0 grade point average and 1400 SAT scores and still not win their support.

Three Key Points to Remember

Creating emotional impact is crucial to your success as a PA school applicant. Personal impact is power—power to achieve whatever you want in your personal life and career. Consider these three key points prior to your interview:

1. **The spoken word is almost the exact opposite of the written word.** The written word is a one-dimensional medium for communicating facts and transferring information. The spoken word, on the other hand, is multi-dimensional and includes a kaleidoscope of nonverbal cues such as posture, eye contact, energy, volume, intonation, and much more. If you want to make an emotional impact and motivate and persuade the admissions committee, you must master the spoken word and learn to make these nonverbal cues work for you rather than against you.

2. **What you say must be believed in order to have impact.** If the committee senses that you are being less than forthright with even one of the questions they ask, you will build a wall of distrust that you probably will not be able to overcome. For your message to be believed, you must be believed.

   I once interviewed a woman who was an accomplished actress. She presented the committee with a very fancy and off-beat resume. Located on the bottom right-hand corner of the resume, below all of her *Off-Broadway* credits, she wrote, *Special Talents: I can tie a cherry stem into a knot with my tongue.* Although this particular talent may be relevant to her role as an actress, it was completely inappropriate for a PA school application and she had already lost her credibility with me and my fellow interviewers before she stepped foot into the interview room. One of my colleagues who wasn't too pleased with the resume notation asked the applicant to comment on her *most memorable patient.* The applicant (actress) started to cry. My colleague asked her, point blank, "How do we know you're not acting now?" The candidate became very silent.

Our *gut feeling* as to whether we like and believe someone is usually based on emotion, not logic. If your voice cracks, or your hands are fidgety, or you cannot make solid eye contact, you'll probably lose credibility with your audience.

3. **Believability is determined at the subconscious level.** Perhaps this is the most important point to remember. How do we determine if we believe someone? Can you build believability out of a mountain of facts and figures? Absolutely not. You cannot even build trust out of a stack of eloquently crafted words. Authoritative credentials, a title, or a letter of recommendation from a "big shot" may give you a little credibility and get you to the interview, but you still have to be believable to "close the sale."

How do you make yourself more believable? First, you must make eye contact. Without good eye contact the committee members may become suspicious of you: What are you hiding? Be sure to smile. Don't become so self-involved and nervous that you forget to relax and smile. Smiling is infectious and will help you and the committee members relax. Use open gestures. Don't sit at the table with your arms folded tightly over your chest. Keep your arms and hands open, which will support the fact that you are an open-minded person. Use a firm handshake. There is nothing worse than a wet, limp handshake. Finally, have good posture and project a strong voice.

Interviewers Are Bombarded with Visual Stimuli that Register at the Preconscious Level

From the moment we walk into the interview, we begin giving off a series of verbal and nonverbal cues. Do you walk into a room tall, or do you slump? Do you have a firm handshake? Do you refer to your patients as "legs" and "arms" or do you refer to them by name? Do you refer to nurses in a derogatory manner, or do you give them the respect they deserve?

An enormous amount of communication is taking place as these thousands of multichannel impressions are carried to the brain. Most of these impressions register at the preconscious level. As a result of these impressions, the brain forms a continuous stream of emotional judgments and assessments. Do I trust this person? Is she honest, evasive, threatening, friendly? Is he interesting, boring, warm, cold, anxious? Is she confident, insecure, or perhaps hiding something?

The emotional judgment that's formed in your preconscious mind about the speaker determines whether you will tune into his or her message or tune out. If you distrust someone at the emotional level, little of what they say will get through.

Getting to Trust

How do we use our natural self to reach the emotional center of our listeners? You've got to be believed in order to be heard. When dealing with the admissions committee, trust and believability are synonymous. You can't have one without the other. To communicate effectively with the committee, you must be trusted. And to win their trust, you must be believable. Belief occurs at the gut level; it's acceptance on faith, it's emotionally based, and it bypasses the intellect.

During the interview, each committee member is sifting through your nuances of behavior. Does your voice quiver, or does it project authority? Do your eyes flicker hesitantly or gaze unflinchingly? Is your posture confident or diffident? These nuances of behavior speak the language of trust.

Who we trust and why, we learned as a baby. One day my son Eddie and I were at the airport in Hartford, Connecticut, on our way to Orlando, Florida to present a seminar. While sitting in the chairs by our gate, we noticed a toddler come playfully strolling over to us with a smile on her face from ear to ear. She was cooing and drooling and having a grand old time. Eddie and I played peek-a-boo with her, causing her to shriek with laughter and excitement. She was a little flirt. Then she suddenly strolled over to a man sitting next to us and smiled playfully at him. Without saying a word, he gave her a look that said, *I'm not interested in you little girl, go away!* The little girl's face went from a huge smile to a little pout. She ran from the man knowing he represented trouble; he wasn't safe.

You cannot communicate with a baby using words. Instead, infants relate to facial expressions, energy, and sound. A baby responds with the same set of verbal cues. The smile is the language of our emotional centers. Even a baby knows that a person who doesn't smile lacks warmth and safety. We learn early in life that the people we should trust are those who (genuinely) smile. To communicate effectively, we must relearn the language of trust.

Did you ever meet someone and instantly like or dislike him, but you didn't know why? When you meet someone for the first time, the emotional center in your brain receives thousands of nonverbal cues that are registered at the preconscious level. Your intuition comes from this; you form an almost immediate impression of that person. You form an impression that is detailed and often richly colored with emotion.

Most candidates approach the interview as though their essay, grades, and SAT scores are what count most. They fail to realize that when they leave that interview, the individual committee members don't comment on logic and reason. Rather, they typically say, "I like her," or "I don't believe him," or "There's something about her that I really like."

Some people can naturally do this without understanding how it works. The candidate who knows how to speak the language of the brain's emotional center—the language of trust—is the candidate most likely to be believed and accepted. That language communicates very rapidly and effectively.

The Likeability Factor

In 1984, President Reagan ran for re-election against Walter Mondale. A Gallup Poll examined three areas with respect to each candidate: 1) issues, 2) party affiliation, 3) likeability. On the issues, the candidates were considered to be dead even. The Democrat clearly had the edge when it

YOU'VE GOT TO BE BELIEVED IN ORDER TO BE HEARD.

came to party affiliation. With respect to likeability, however, Reagan had the edge and won the election. It was the personality factor that dominated.

As applicants, we pride ourselves on having a great grade point average, 1400 SAT scores, and years of hands-on medical experience. But when it's time to interview, it's your likeability that determines whether you receive a letter of acceptance or a letter of rejection. As soon as you walk into that interview room, it's the visual connection that sets the beginning of trust and believability.

The Eye Factor

The eye is the only sensory organ that contains brain cells. Memory experts invariably link the objects they remember to a visual image. Research shows that it's the visual image that makes the greatest impact in communication.

The spoken message is made up of only three components:

- ▶ The **verbal** component
- ▶ The **vocal** component
- ▶ The **visual** component

A few years ago, a prominent UCLA professor conducted a landmark study on the relationship of the three components of the spoken word. He measured the effect of each of these three components on the believability of the spoken message. The **verbal** message, or the actual words that we use, are what most people concentrate on, but this is actually the most insignificant part of the spoken message. The **vocal** component is made up of the intonation, projection, and resonance of your spoken message. It is the **visual** message, however, the emotion and expression of your body and face as you speak, that carries the most weight.

This professor also found that the degree of consistency or inconsistency between these three key elements is the factor that determines the believability of your message. The more these three factors harmonize, the more believable you are as a candidate. If your verbal message is not in harmony with your body language, you send a mixed signal to the emotional center of the other person's brain. Your message may or may not get through to the decision-making, rational portion of the brain. The three components of the spoken message are quantified as follows:

- ▶ Verbal = 7%
- ▶ Voice = 38%
- ▶ Visual = 55%

In other words, what you see is what you get. If you come into the interview room yawning or dressed inappropriately, nothing you do or say will help you. The interviewer is likely to shut you out immediately and not hear a word you have to say.

HOW DO YOU ENHANCE YOUR MESSAGE?

The first way to enhance your communication is with eye contact. This is the number-one skill you should develop prior to interviewing. The three rules and exercises for maintaining eye contact are as follows:

IT IS THE **VISUAL** MESSAGE, HOWEVER, THE EMOTION AND EXPRESSION OF YOUR BODY AND FACE AS YOU SPEAK, THAT CARRIES THE MOST WEIGHT.

THE FIRST WAY TO ENHANCE YOUR COMMUNICATION IS WITH EYE CONTACT. THIS IS THE NUMBER-ONE SKILL YOU SHOULD DEVELOP PRIOR TO INTERVIEWING.

Rules

1. Use involvement rather than intimacy or intimidation.
2. Count to five (involvement), then look away.
3. Don't dart your eyes; this represents a lack of confidence.

Exercises

1. **Use video feedback**. Tape yourself speaking with someone and watch for your use of, or violation of, the above three rules.
2. **Practice one-on-one**. Have a conversation with someone you trust and ask this person for direct feedback with respect to these rules.
3. **Practice with a paper audience**. Place Post-it Notes with smiling faces drawn on them on a chair and practice making eye contact, counting to five and looking away.

The next way to enhance your message is with posture and movement. A good posture commands attention, and movement shows confidence. Walk into the room standing tall. Don't slump. When you speak to your interviewer, don't be afraid to add movement to your message. You don't have to wave your hands all over the room, but use open gestures to come across as a friendly, open-minded person.

Rules

1. Stand tall.
2. Watch your lower body; don't lean back on one hip or rock back and forth.
3. Get in the ready position; lean slightly forward if you're sitting, or on the balls of your feet if you're standing.
4. Use movement to show that you're excited, enthusiastic, and confident.

Exercises

1. **Walk away from the wall**. Stand with your back against a wall, heels pressed against the wall along with your head, neck, and shoulders. Try to push the small of your back into the wall. Now simply walk away from the wall and feel how upright and correct your posture becomes. Try to shake off this posture; you can't. Practice this exercise daily so that when you walk into the interview room, you'll command attention.
2. **Use the ready position**. Remember, if you're standing, sit up slightly on the balls of your feet. If you are sitting, lean slightly forward toward your interviewer(s).
3. **Use a paper audience**.

The third way to enhance your message is with dress and appearance. You only get two seconds to make your initial impression on your interviewers. If you blow it, it may take over thirty minutes to recover, and most interviews only last for twenty minutes. So, it is critical to make a good first impression.

When you are dressed up for an interview, only 10% of your skin is showing. Be sure that your face is well shaven or your make-up is not too overbearing. Comb/style your hair, avoid wearing extravagant jewelry, clean and trim your nails, and use cologne/perfume sparingly.

A GOOD POSTURE COMMANDS ATTENTION, AND MOVEMENT SHOWS CONFIDENCE.

YOU ONLY GET TWO SECONDS TO MAKE YOUR INITIAL IMPRESSION ON YOUR INTERVIEWERS.

Rules

1. Be appropriate; *When in Rome . . .*
2. Be conservative; when in doubt, dress up.
3. Men, always button your jacket.
4. Don't overkill perfume or cologne.
5. Always bring a small mirror and check your face before interviewing.

Exercises

1. **Get people feedback.** Ask friends and relatives how well you present yourself. Be open to constructive criticism.
2. **Be observant; read fashion magazines.** Find a style with which you are comfortable. Don't go over the edge, however.

The final way to enhance your message is with gestures and your smile. Do you speak with conviction, enthusiasm, and passion? Are you friendly or stuffy? Do you speak with open gestures and a warm smile, or are you a "fig leaf flasher," always covering and uncovering your groin with your hands. Remember, openness equals likeability.

Rules

1. Be aware of nervous gestures and stop them.
2. Lift your apples—smile. Make believe that you have apples on your cheekbones and try to lift them up to your forehead.
3. Feel your smile.
4. Caution: Phony smiles don't work.

Exercises

1. **Imitate someone whom you feel is an effective communicator and play the part with gusto.** Get used to using open gestures and expressions.
2. **Be natural.** Incorporate some of these gestures into your daily communication.

THE ENERGY FACTOR

Energy is the fuel that drives the car to success. You don't want to run out of gas when you're halfway up the hill. Think back to the last morning that you awoke feeling completely refreshed, like you could conquer the world. Wasn't that a powerful space to be in? This is exactly where you need to be on the day of the interview—in the *zone*. This next section focuses on ways to unlock your inner energy and present yourself in the best light to the admissions committee.

Voice and Vocal Variety

Use intonation and inflection in your voice. Speaking in a monotone can be deadly and put your listeners to sleep. Observe and practice the following rules and exercises to add energy to your voice.

Rules

1. Make your voice naturally authoritative; speak from the diaphragm.
2. Put your voice on a roller coaster; practice reading from magazines using intonation and inflection.

3. Be aware of your telephone voice; it represents 84% of the emotional impact when people can't see you.
4. Smile when talking on the telephone; people can feel your smile right through the phone.
5. Put your real feelings into your voice.

Exercises

1. **Breathe from the diaphragm.** Take in a deep breath from your nose and let it out slowly, stopping to feel the pressure on your diaphragm. This is where a strong voice originates.
2. **Project your voice.** Try speaking in a normal voice first, then project your voice so it reaches the back of the room. Try to find the right depth in your voice without straining your vocal chords.
3. **Practice varying your pitch and pace.** Read from magazines.

Words and Nonwords

Energize with words and avoid using nonwords that are meaningless and take away from your message.

Rules

1. Build your vocabulary, especially with synonyms. I provide you with a list of synonyms in Appendix D.
2. Paint word pictures. Create motion and emotion with metaphors.
3. Beware of jargon, especially medical jargon. Use "operating room" instead of "O.R."
4. Avoid meaningless nonwords like *ahh, uhm, so, well,* and *you know.* Replace these nonwords with a pause. A properly timed pause adds drama, energy, and power to your message. Try listening to the voice of the famous commentator, Paul Harvey. He is the master of the pause and has made a career out of using this technique.

Listener Involvement

Humans communicate, and books dispense information. Try using the following techniques to add an extra punch to your communication.

Rules

1. Use a strong opening. Make it visual and energetic by including pauses, action and motion, and joy and laughter.
2. Maintain eye communication. When you enter the room for a group interview, survey your listeners for 3 to 5 seconds, gauge, and adjust.
3. Lean toward your listeners.
4. Create interest by maintaining eye contact and having high energy.

Use Humor Effectively

"I will not make age an issue in this campaign. I will not exploit my opponent's youth and inexperience." These words changed an entire campaign in Ronald Reagan's favor, after he spoke them at a national debate with Walter Mondale. In reference to an *age* question he anticipated he would be asked, Reagan was prepared with this witty response, which turned out to be the most remembered sentences uttered at the debate.

I do not recommend that you tell jokes at your interview; however, remember, fun is better than funny. The goal is not comedy, but connection. Find the form of humor that works for you, and be natural.

KARIN'S EXPERIENCE:

Before we start the next chapter, which covers an overview of the actual interview process, let's take a look at what one of my friends and colleagues has to say about her interview experience at Yale University. Karin did not get accepted the first year she applied, however, after making some adjustments, she re-applied the next year, and was accepted. Her experience offers a great deal of insight into the interview process.

Applying to PA school or any other graduate school can be a very stressful process. Knowing yourself and the profession you are striving to enter are two of the most important factors in the application process. This is particularly evident during the interview. Being absolutely sure that a career as a physician assistant is what you truly desire, you must have an in-depth and intimate knowledge of what a physician assistant does. Conveying this knowledge and your passion for the profession to the interviewer will translate to a successful interview.

When applying to PA school, an impressive application is always important. Once an interview is granted, demonstrating your attributes in person is even more important. The interviewers are looking for someone with strong character, good communication skills, and focused goals. Even with mediocre qualifications on paper, an impressive interview can significantly increase your chances of being accepted.

My first attempt at PA school proved to be a painful eye-opener. After graduating from one of the top five schools in the country, earning a B.A. in biology, I was convinced a career in research as a PhD was my calling in life. After several months working in a cell biology laboratory, I realized this was not my life dream. I soon began volunteering at a university emergency department, where I first encountered a physician assistant. Immediately, I knew this career path was one that I would enjoy and I began preparing to enter PA school. I filled out all of the applications and mentally began to prepare for the interviews. During this year of preparation, I also became engaged to my current husband and found myself preparing for a wedding. As you can imagine, the year was quite hectic and emotionally overwhelming. One by one I heard from each of the schools, and to my utter surprise, I was rejected by all of them. I could not believe it. What had happened? After the initial shock subsided, I soon realized why I was denied acceptance.

Despite being physically present at the various interviews, I was not present in spirit. Besides being distracted by my wedding plans, I had not fully let go of the idea of a career in research. The following year, I not only had to deal with a bruised ego, but I was also forced to take a long, hard look at myself. I continued doing research and volunteering in the emergency department. I decided to start shadowing a PA and realized I had a lot more to learn about the profession. I quickly embraced the idea that, yes, I wanted to be a PA. I focused my energy on improving myself as an applicant. As a result, I was accepted to my school of choice. I completed the program in two years, finishing second in my class.

Whatever your goals are in life, you must embrace them fully. This is what I learned during my application and interview process. This is exactly what went wrong the first year I applied. Understanding your individual

KNOWING YOURSELF AND THE PROFESSION YOU ARE STRIVING TO ENTER ARE TWO OF THE MOST IMPORTANT FACTORS IN THE APPLICATION PROCESS.

THE INTERVIEWERS ARE LOOKING FOR SOMEONE WITH STRONG CHARACTER, GOOD COMMUNICATION SKILLS, AND FOCUSED GOALS.

WHATEVER YOUR GOALS ARE IN LIFE, YOU MUST EMBRACE THEM FULLY.

THE INTERVIEW (PART ONE)

strengths and weaknesses and improving upon them are an excellent way to make you a stronger applicant. Learning as much as you can about physician assistants and how you as an individual will satisfy your dreams is as important to your interview as it is to your lifelong happiness.

Karin Augur, PA-C

The Interview
(Part Two)

This chapter will cover an overview of the interview process and give you a feel for what to expect. In addition, I will provide you with 21 tips to help you excel at your interview.

OVERVIEW OF THE INTERVIEW PROCESS

Not all interviews are conducted in the same fashion. The following represents only a sample of what you may face on interview day.

When you get up on the morning of your interview, and before you even get out of bed, ask yourself this question: *What is the worst thing that could possibly happen today?* Once you think about the answer to this question, and accept the fact that you will still have your life, health, and family, you will feel more relaxed and be able to perform to your potential.

Once you arrive at the interview location, someone from the PA program staff will greet you. Whoever that person is, be sure to smile, shake hands, and be polite. You are now officially being evaluated, and this process will continue until you leave in the afternoon or evening.

You will be directed to a room where the other interviewees will be seated (unless you're the first to arrive, of course). Again, you should smile, offer your hand to shake, and introduce yourself to everyone. Even if someone walks in after you, be the first to extend a handshake and a hello. Remember, you are being evaluated all day, and this is a good way to show off some of your good qualities.

It is a good idea to speak with everyone—ask them about their background, where else they have interviewed, where they are from, etc. Allow others to speak, too. The key is not being too shy or obnoxious. Find the balance, and, above all, be genuine.

After everyone arrives, you will begin a short series of talks with the Director of the Program, the Director of Admissions, and the Financial Aid Officer. Listen intently, ask intelligent questions, and stay relaxed. Do not feel that you have to dominate the situation; you'll have time to shine when the actual interviews start.

Next up are the case scenarios. These are a set of three to four written questions that you will all have about fifteen minutes to answer. They are not meant to stress you out before the interview, but are simply a way to get an idea of your ability to reason and make sound judgments.

Once you've finished the case scenarios, you'll be split up into two groups; half of you will begin the interview process, and half of you will attend a class with the first-year students. When you go to the class, remember that you are always being evaluated. Inappropriate comments to students can ruin your day. Pay attention to the lecture, remember the instructor's name, and only ask sensible, relevant questions if you feel it is absolutely necessary. If you like, you may ask the students questions before and after the class.

At most programs, the interviews consist of three parts: the student interview, the group interview, and the single interview. There are usually two students, a first year and a second year, in the student interview. The group interview consists of three PAs or MDs, and the single interviewer is usually the senior PA or a psychologist/psychiatrist. **Please keep in mind that not all programs follow the same interview patterns or procedures.**

After the morning interviews, you will have lunch, meet with some of the current students, and then switch roles with the other applicants. If you have already interviewed, do not make any comments about the questions or process.

At the end of the day you will all be offered a tour of the facility. We recommend that you take this tour unless you have a flight or train to catch. If that's the case, let the Dean know that you have to keep to your schedule, and thank him or her for the opportunity to interview. If you go on the tour, ask intelligent questions, don't fool around, and most importantly, ask yourself is this the kind of place where you'd like to go to school.

THE STUDENT INTERVIEW

Although this tends to be the most relaxed interview, let your guard down and you could find yourself re-applying next year. The students take this interview very seriously, and they could make you or break you. The usually do not have access to all of your application, but they will score you and comment on your performance. They basically want to know three things about you:

1. Do you know what a PA is and does?
2. Have you worked as hard as they have to get here?
3. Would you make a good classmate?

Keep in mind that students tend to grade tougher than the committee members. Remember in grade school when the teacher allowed the students to grade their own papers? We're much tougher on ourselves. Students have a great sense of pride in their accomplishments, their school, and the PA profession. Don't blow it by making comments like, "You're only students" or "The hard part is over; you guys will be easy." You might as well say goodbye now.

A good tip is to ask the students what they like about the program and why they like it. Ask them why you should pick this school, if given the opportunity, over Duke, Yale, or Emory, for example. Let them sell you a little bit.

THE GROUP INTERVIEW

For some, this is the toughest part of the day. I've seen applicants cry, get mad, clam up, shake, rattle, and roll in this interview. In this one you usually

PLEASE KEEP IN MIND THAT NOT ALL PROGRAMS FOLLOW THE SAME INTERVIEW PATTERNS OR PROCEDURES.

ALTHOUGH THIS TENDS TO BE THE MOST RELAXED INTERVIEW, LET YOUR GUARD DOWN AND YOU COULD FIND YOURSELF RE-APPLYING NEXT YEAR.

have three or more committee members, usually PAs and MDs, who have just re-read your application and have specific and general questions in mind. The committee has six basic things to find out from you:

1. Do you have a good concept of the PA profession?
2. Can you handle this program academically?
3. Will you *fit in* with the class, and will you be able to contribute to it?
4. Are you a compassionate person?
5. Are you a team player?
6. Can you handle the stress of the program?

It is your job to convince the group that the answer is *yes* on all accounts. We will cover the questions, and specific answers, in the next chapter.

The group has no hidden agenda; they're really not trying to trip you up. Some applicants become very defensive when asked certain questions. Remain cool, never raise your voice, and, as the commercial says, *never let them see you sweat*. The committee wants you to do well; some of these people may have even originally scored your application to get you here.

The following are some general tips for interviewing:

▶ Be honest.
▶ Be genuine.
▶ If you don't know the answer, admit it.
▶ Don't beg to be accepted.
▶ Think! Think! Think!
▶ Smile.
▶ Make eye contact.

Once the committee interview is over, you'll be asked if you have any questions. See the end of the chapter for a short list of appropriate questions to ask the committee. You do not have to ask questions. In fact, the committee will not care one way or the other if you ask questions or not. The exception is asking too many questions at the interview, or asking inappropriate questions.

Before you leave the room, be sure to thank each member of the group by name.

THE INDIVIDUAL INTERVIEW

The purpose of this interview is threefold:

1. To verify what you have told the other interviewers.
2. To see if your answers are consistent.
3. To find out more about your personal life.

Please be consistent with your answers. If you have done your homework, you'll have no problem. For instance, don't think that you can tell the students and the group interviewers that you never thought of going to medical school, and then confide in the single interviewer that you applied twice but weren't accepted. This is inconsistent and may lower your score.

If you draw a psychologist for your single interview, he/she may ask you very personal questions. Don't get flustered. Don't volunteer too much information either. Avoid talking about drugs, sexual preference, the family alcoholic, and topics that may get you into trouble. If they hand you a rope, don't hang yourself with it.

BEFORE YOU LEAVE THE ROOM, BE SURE TO THANK EACH MEMBER OF THE GROUP BY NAME.

SCORING/RATING YOUR INTERVIEW

After each interview session, morning and afternoon, the entire committee meets to discuss the candidates, compare notes, and give you a score. You may be rated in six areas; within these, each committee may decide on common indicators that best summarize the qualities of a good PA.

1. Cognitive/Verbal Ability

The committee will want to know if you have the ability to think through a problem and respond appropriately. Are you a lifelong learner? Can you articulate your ideas in a logical sequence? How perceptive are you about others? Here, both verbal ability and written skills are important indicators. The committee will also want to see evidence of your organizational skills, for instance, time-management strategies, or your ability to prioritize, and indeed your problem-solving processes. You will need to show too that you understand the rigor of the PA program of study.

2. Motivation to Become a PA

Are you strongly motivated or just testing the waters? Why do you want to become a PA? Are you interested in patients or the science of medicine? The committee will want to get a sense of your enthusiasm and commitment to the profession. You will need to demonstrate that you are a practical person who has had experience with patient care.

3. Understanding of the PA Profession

Do you know what PA practice entails? Do you know any PAs? Have you worked with any PAs? In this area, the committee will be looking to see if you are realistic in your understanding of the role of a PA and that you also have a positive attitude toward RNs/MDs. Once again, the committee will be interested in how patient-oriented you are.

4. Interpersonal Skills/Behavior

Do you work collaboratively? Would you be respected by patients and colleagues? Or do you come across as too eager and domineering? Are you courteous and tactful in dealing with others? Are you compassionate? There is a range of key areas within this category, from good grooming and personal presentation to more complex communication skills, where the panel will be looking to see that you demonstrate appropriate listening skills, have an understanding of different audiences, are warm and open without being overly friendly, and can be diplomatic when required. Obviously, coming across as too aggressive or fabricating your experience to win points are not indicators a panel would want to find.

5. Ability to Handle Stress

Except for a little anxiety, can you relax and be at ease? Do you have a sense of humor? Are you articulate? Do you convey your ideas clearly? Do you remain poised and relatively calm in the face of stressful situations? Do you have a measure of self-possession? Are you over-anxious or confused in times of stress?

6. Personal Characteristics

Are you thoughtful and innovative? Are you a technician or a decision maker? Are the facts you present in your interview consistent with your written file? Some of the key areas that a panel may look for here are your level of maturity, self-drive, and determination, balanced with how flexible and creative you may be. Your ability to empathize with others will also be an important indicator in this area.

Each program has its own rating system. For instance, a scale of 1–10 may be used, with 10 being the best (accept) and 1 being the worst (reject); or a scale that places applicants in one of the following categories: *Definite Acceptance, Probable Acceptance, Uncertain, Probable Rejection, Definite Rejection.* After each session of interviews is over, the committee meets in one room to give the final scores. An applicant's name will be called, and each committee member will simply call out his or her score. Once the scores are collected on all of the applicants, the discussions begin. Again, each program has its own method of evaluating interviewees.

If an applicant scores all 1s or all 10s, there's nothing to discuss. Most applicants, however, fall somewhere in the middle and require further discussion. For instance, if the students score an applicant 10 and 10, respectively; the group scores the applicant 10, 8, and 10, respectively; and the single interviewer scores the same applicant 4, there's obviously a problem here. What does the single interviewer know that the rest of the committee doesn't?

Upon asking the single interviewer, we may find out that everything went well until the applicant mentioned his problems with drugs and alcohol. There is a problem. At this point, the students and group change their scores and the applicant does not get in.

The process can also work in reverse. Someone may really champion an applicant and convince everyone else to give a better score. There is an extensive number of checks and balances set up to be sure that only the best candidates get accepted.

INTERVIEWING TIPS/RULES

1. Arrive to the interview on time.
2. Dress appropriately. Men: suit and tie; Women: business suit; shined shoes
3. Bring a compact mirror to quickly look over your face.
4. Smile genuinely.
5. Always offer your (firm) handshake first.
6. Look everyone in the eyes.
7. Speak clearly and loudly enough to be heard.
8. Use proper English.
9. Say "please" and "thank you."
10. Don't sit until asked to do so.
11. Bring a copy of your entire application; review it when you have free time.
12. Prepare a short list of good questions to ask.
13. Bring a picture of yourself.
14. When interviewing, try not to make nervous hand movements.
15. Don't become defensive.
16. Don't ever raise your voice.
17. Don't say too much.
18. Listen to everyone with genuine interest.

19. Be consistent.
20. Answer the question briefly.
21. Don't ramble.

GOOD QUESTIONS TO ASK

After you finish each interview, you will be given the opportunity to ask questions. You do not have to ask any questions, and if you don't, it won't be counted against you. But if you ask inappropriate questions, or too many questions, you're liable to annoy the interviewer(s). If you choose not to ask any questions, simply say, "No thank you. I've had all of my questions answered already." If you do ask questions, use the following list as a guide.

Ask Students:

▶ What do you like best about this program?
▶ Why should I pick this program over any other program?
▶ What do you like least about this program?

Ask the Group:

▶ If I'm selected, why should I pick this program over Duke or George Washington?
▶ What is this school's **first-time** pass/fail rate on the national boards?
▶ What is the highlight of this program?

Ask the Single Interviewer:

▶ Why is this program so successful?
▶ What can be improved about this program?
▶ What is this school's **first-time** pass/fail rate on the boards?

Do Not Ask:

▶ So, what do you do for excitement?
▶ How's the partying around here?
▶ Are there lots of women/men here?

These are inappropriate questions to ask an interviewer.

AFTER THE INTERVIEW

After you go home from the interview, write a letter of thanks to the director of the program. This will be placed in your file, whether you get in or not, and if it's the latter, it may help you next year.

AFTER YOU GO HOME FROM THE INTERVIEW, WRITE A LETTER OF THANKS TO THE DIRECTOR OF THE PROGRAM.

The Interview
(Part Three)

In our last chapter we focused on the interview process and the particular skills you must exhibit to perform well. In this chapter we will focus on the exact questions that you are likely to be asked, and I will provide you with an insider's slant on what the committee really wants to know.

Too many applicants feel that they can come to the interview and just wing it. This can be a fatal mistake. In this climate of hundreds of applicants for too few slots, you must practice, practice, practice. If you don't, you may find yourself applying again next year.

I do not recommend that you memorize the exact answers to the questions I give here. This, too, can be a fatal mistake. Rather, I encourage you to incorporate these concepts into your own experiences and formulate answers that are specific to you and your situation.

The questions and answers will be set up in this format:

▶ Question:
▶ In other words:
▶ Answer:

I will first give you the question. Then I will tell you what the question really asks for. Finally, I will give an appropriate response. The first six areas will cover those discussed in the last chapter, Scoring/Rating Your Interview. The remainder are more questions that you could very likely be asked. Keep your answers short but concise.

COGNITIVE/VERBAL ABILITY

Question: How has your academic work prepared you for the PA profession?

In other words: Can you handle the rigor of our didactic phase?

Answer: If you have filled out the worksheets from Chapter 6, you will be well prepared to answer this one. "I have a B.S. in chemistry with a 3.3 GPA. In addition, I recently completed a microbiology course and anatomy and physiology, receiving an A in each class. Throughout college, I worked at a part-time job and volunteered at the local hospital."

This applicant not only demonstrates the ability to handle difficult science course work; she also demonstrates good time management skills and the ability to do more than one thing at a given time.

TOO MANY APPLICANTS FEEL THAT THEY CAN COME TO THE INTERVIEW AND JUST WING IT. THIS CAN BE A FATAL MISTAKE.

Question: Tell us about the last book you read.

In other words: Tell us something about yourself—your interests.

Answer: You may not want to mention that you read the latest Danielle Steele novel. Play it safe: "I just read the autobiography of Abraham Lincoln. He surmounted incredible odds to become the President. It was a very inspiring story."

Question: What is the most important issue facing the health care system in the United States?

In other words: Can you articulate an intelligent response to an area that affects all of us as citizens and as health care workers?

Answer: Read the journals recommended throughout this text. When reading the newspaper, focus on these issues, which are written about every day. Talk to other PAs and get a sense for what's going on in this arena. How does it affect them?

"I feel that 'managed care' is an important concern at this time. Some providers feel that the insurance companies are now dictating how long a patient can remain in the hospital for a given illness. For example, until recently, mothers were allowed only one day in the hospital after having a baby, so-called drive-by deliveries. On the other hand, however, we must do something with respect to excessive health care costs. It's a real dilemma."

MOTIVATION TO BECOME A PA

Question: Why do you want to be a PA?

In other words: Have you thought about this intelligently?

Answer: You must answer this question in 250 words or less and provide an answer that shows insight and enthusiasm.

> YOU MUST ANSWER THIS QUESTION IN 250 WORDS OR LESS AND PROVIDE AN ANSWER THAT SHOWS INSIGHT AND ENTHUSIASM.

"After serving as a hospital corpsman for four years and an emergency room technician for one year, I realized that I found a niche in health care. I enjoy providing comfort to patients and placing them at ease. I also enjoy being a member of the team and doing my part to provide the best quality of care to the patient.

"I want to do more, however. I would like to be able to diagnose and treat patients as well. Although I love my current job, I feel that I could contribute much more in this newly enhanced role as a PA.

"I have thought about medical school; however, I have a family and I do not have the time, nor the inclination, to spend the next eight or so years of my life pursuing that goal. From what I have experienced, PAs have a challenging and rewarding role in the health care system. I have never met a PA who disliked his or her job.

"I simply want to practice medicine. I rather like the fact that PAs have physicians available for consultation with difficult presentations. I feel no need to be independent, although I think in situations I'll be somewhat autonomous. This is why I prefer becoming a PA rather than a nurse practitioner, who frequently practices independently.

"Finally, I like the fact that PAs are trained in the medical model, in contrast to nursing, and that they can move from one specialty to the next without having to retrain. This is a benefit not even afforded the MD."

In less than 250 words, the applicant has managed to answer several questions here and touch on several key points:

▶ Demonstrates experience
▶ Teamwork
▶ Enthusiasm
▶ Why not an MD?
▶ Why not a nurse practitioner?
▶ Why not a nurse?
▶ Understands dependent practitioner role
▶ Realizes may still be autonomous

Question: Have you applied to other programs?

In other words: 1) How serious are you? 2) What's your logic in choosing the programs you have?

Answer: By applying to other programs, you show that you want to become a PA and you are maximizing your chances of getting into school. In addition, you should be prepared to discuss why you selected the programs you have.

WHAT'S YOUR LOGIC IN CHOOSING THE PROGRAMS YOU HAVE?

"I applied to Northeastern, Quinnipiac, and Duke because they offer a master's degree."

"I applied to Yale, Quinnipiac, Northeastern, and Springfield College because my wife will be supporting me and our children, and if we have to move, she may not be able to find a job that pays enough to cover the rent and put food on the table."

"I applied to Cornell, Alabama, and Cuyahoga because I'm really interested in doing surgery."

(Note: Your transcripts from the various colleges frequently list the other programs to which you've applied. So, many times the committee knows where else you've applied.)

Question: What have you done to prepare yourself for this profession?

In other words: Are you a serious applicant or just testing the waters because you're not happy with your current profession?

Answer: Review your worksheets and list all of your preparation and accomplishments to get you here today.

"In addition to my degree in biology, I also worked as a nurse's aide for three years. Recently, I went back to night school to take courses in cell biology and pharmacology. In addition, I have volunteered at the local hospital's HIV clinic for the past six months.

"I have also shadowed two PAs this year; one works in internal medicine and the other works in OB-GYN. And, I have joined the AAPA and ConnAPA to keep up with current issues facing the profession."

Don't fabricate here. Hopefully, you have done something to prepare yourself for getting into PA school.

Question: Have you done anything to increase your chances of being accepted to the PA program?

In other words: This is especially important for re-applicants. Just how serious and committed are you? What makes you stand out from the person sitting next to you this morning?

WHAT MAKES YOU STAND OUT FROM THE PERSON SITTING NEXT TO YOU THIS MORNING?

Answer: This is your opportunity to shine. Tell the committee about all of the PAs you have contacted, shadowed, and communicated with. Tell them about the recent courses you've completed and all of your health care experience. Point out that you have joined your state Academy of Physician Assistants and the American Academy of Physician Assistants. Let them know, by name, any and all of their current students that you have worked with. In other words, demonstrate that getting into PA school has been your mission for the past twelve months.

UNDERSTANDING OF THE PA PROFESSION

Question: What is your understanding of what PAs do?

In other words: Are you aware of the PA concept?

DO NOT RECITE THE AAPA DEFINITION OF A PA HERE. PERSONALIZE YOUR ANSWER BASED ON YOUR EXPERIENCE WITH PAs.

Answer: Do not recite the AAPA definition of a PA here. Personalize your answer based on your experience with PAs. If you have no experience with PAs, then don't try to fool the committee into thinking you do; you'll be caught. You may want to start with, "From my understanding . . ." Otherwise, give your understanding of the profession based on first-hand knowledge:

"Based on my experience as a technician in the emergency room, and through my recent shadowing of two PAs, I have observed several PAs in action. Most of them work autonomously but usually have the availability of a physician when needed. In the ER the PAs are usually the first to see the patients when they arrive. They take a short history from the patient or EMTs, perform a physical exam, and order the appropriate tests. At times, they suture, apply casts, or perform various other procedures.

"The internal medicine PAs are part of a team, working closely with other students, interns, residents, and the attending physician. They often round with the team and present and discuss their patients. They also report to the ER to interview their patients, write the H&P, order the appropriate tests, and formulate the initial plan."

This applicant is explaining, from personal experience, the role of the PA at her institution. This is much better than giving the AAPA definition of the profession, and, believe me, many people will simply cite this definition instead of personalizing their answer.

Question: Tell us about the role you see the PA playing in the health care system.

In other words: Are you familiar with the PA concept?

ARE YOU FAMILIAR WITH THE PA CONCEPT?

Answer: This is similar to the above question but with a little twist. Do not mention a hierarchy here of physician, PA, nurse, etc. Keep the focus on teamwork. "PAs are a part of the health care team, working with physicians, nurses, and other members to provide the best care to the patient."

Question: How do you feel about taking call or working 60 or more hours per week as a second-year student?

In other words: Do you know what you're getting yourself into?

Answer: You may be asking about now, *But I thought PAs didn't have to work like interns, putting in so many hours?* While you may choose not to work so many hours as a PA, when you are a PA student and on rotation, you are expected to work as many hours as the medical student or intern. The correct response would be, "I'm prepared to do whatever it takes to be a PA. I have spoken with several PA students, and I know what I am up against. I welcome the challenge of learning all that I can while I'm in school."

INTERPERSONAL SKILLS/BEHAVIOR

Question: Describe an interaction you have had with a patient that made an impact on you.

In other words: Do you have compassion or are you simply science-oriented, more interested in the pathology than the patient?

Answer: Be prepared to discuss a patient who has made an impact on you in some way. Let the committee know what the situation was, how the patient made out, and what you've learned from him/her.

"My first trauma patient was a 23-year-old Portuguese gentleman who was involved in an industrial fire. He spoke no English. I remember the burn team coming to the ER and assessing him. He appeared to be in no pain, even though he was burned over most of his body. I originally thought he was wearing gloves, until someone pointed out that was his skin hanging from his hands.

"The burn team assessed the patient, left the room, and began drawing figures on a piece of paper. They concluded that the man had less than a 3% chance of surviving. They went back into the trauma room, this time with an interpreter, and explained the situation to the patient. They asked him if he wanted them to operate, which would be extremely painful, or simply make him comfortable. I remember his response was to operate. What else would a 23-year-old say, I thought?

"The patient died after surgery, but I will never forget him, and how he must have felt lying on the trauma room table, not understanding English, and having someone ask if he preferred to live in pain or die?"

Question: What do you think is the most difficult situation described in the interview scenarios that you completed earlier today? Why?

In other words: Do you have any hidden feelings about AIDS patients, psychiatric patients, or drug addicts?

Answer: Don't shoot yourself in the foot. Hopefully, you did not give any controversial answers, as suggested. You can simply reply, in response to the trauma patient with HIV: "Every day I witness staff members in the hospital not taking universal precautions by wearing gloves or protective eyewear. I do my best to lead by example and always protect myself, but I must admit that I cringe when I see others take universal precautions so lightly."

This response shifts the focus off the HIV-positive patient and concentrates on the issue of universal precautions.

ABILITY TO HANDLE STRESS

Question: Describe the most stressful work or academic situation you have been in, and tell us how you dealt with it.

In other words: What constitutes stress to you, and do you know how to cope with stress?

Answer: The committee knows that interviewing for PA school is stressful enough, and they probably have a good idea of your ability to handle it at this point. But give them a little more insight by example:

"I find the best way to deal with stress is to avoid it! But we all know that isn't always possible. My most stressful situation came as a junior officer in the Air Force. I was placed in charge of a bomb clean-up operation at Nellis Air Force base in Nevada. I had forty people working for me—carpenters, explosive ordnance disposal people, and several truck drivers. The range we were cleaning was used by F-16 pilots to practice bombing skills. We had to sweep the range, remove the live ordnance that remained, and build new targets. Under each old piece of plywood we found a rattlesnake. Between the bombs and the snakes, I was never so scared in my life; and I was in charge!

"To get through this situation, I relied on the senior noncommissioned officers from each group. Each morning we'd meet and make a plan of action. We kept in contact via radio all day. I'm proud to say that we had no casualties, and we all received a letter of commendation from our commanding officer. Teamwork got us through."

Although this is a dramatic story, for which most of us have no similar experience, the applicant explained that he relied on others' help to get everyone through the situation. He used teamwork and planning each day to get through.

By the way, providing a copy of the letter of commendation in your application will provide verification for your statement.

Question: How do you usually deal with stress?

In other words: Do you have any stress-relieving activities? Some interviewers may also ask this question to see if you exercise.

Answer: I recommend that you take up some form of exercise for your own good. Then you can answer, "I run three miles a day."

Question: What kind of personal stress do you see associated with our PA program?

In other words: Do you have a realistic view of the rigor of the program? Do you have any hidden fears about coming here to school?

Answer: "After speaking to several of your students, both first year and second year, I am aware of how difficult the two years will be. For instance, I know that the didactic phase is extremely comprehensive and fast paced. In addition, I'm aware of the amount of hours I'll be expected to put in on clinical rotations. However, I am confident that my previous college work in chemistry and biology has prepared me well for further study, and I have never been afraid to roll up my sleeves and work long, hard hours. I look forward to the challenge."

Question: What kind of stress do you see associated with the PA profession?

In other words: Are you aware of how far the profession has come and what challenges we still have ahead?

Answer: "The PA profession has come a long way in a short time. I know that the early PAs had to fight for all of the respect and privileges that everyone enjoys today. On the other hand, there are still issues to be resolved and more work to be done. Some nurses and nurse practitioners take issue with the scope of PA practice; a case in point is in Mississippi. We will always face new challenges, especially with health care reform, but the profession has come too far, and if PAs continue doing as well as they have done in the past, the profession will continue to grow."

PERSONAL CHARACTERISTICS

Question: What do you do outside of work or academic studies?

In other words: Are you a well-rounded person?

Answer: Go back to your worksheets in Chapter 6 and make a list of your extracurricular activities. List things you like to do: biking, hiking, running, investing, playing in a band, etc.

Question: Please discuss your answer to question #___ on the interview questionnaire. Or, What did you mean by ___ on your essay?

In other words: Can you think on your feet?

Answer: As mentioned already, the best way to deal with stress is to avoid it. Don't write anything controversial on your questionnaire or narrative and you'll never have to answer a question like this. But if you do, keep your cool, take a deep breath, and answer the question to the best of your ability. Don't add insult to injury by arguing your point. Perhaps you misunderstood the original question.

Question: Your file indicates that you have had difficulty with ___(e.g., time management or science course work). Would you like to explain this?

In other words: Have you thought about your shortcomings? What have you done to change things?

Answer: Of course, you would like to comment. You have hopefully anticipated this question about your grades in high school, or why you flunked freshman chemistry in college. "In high school I had no real focus in life and I simply wanted to graduate. After working for Dr. Smith and realizing I loved medicine, I went to college with a purpose, to get into PA school, and my grades improved tremendously."

Question: What accommodations, if any, do you need to successfully complete this program?

In other words: Is there any part of the program you will not participate in?

Answer: We had several women in our class who weren't thrilled with the idea of classmates doing breast exams on one another. This issue came up at the beginning of our physical exam sessions. It caused a lot of stress for the class and the students involved. If you feel strongly about an issue, with respect to the program, discuss it before you begin the program, but not necessarily at the interview.

MORE INTERVIEW QUESTIONS

The following questions may or may not be similar to the above. Keep in mind that specific examples and vignettes make for better answers than a simple yes or no. By the same token, keep your answers very brief, but concise.

ARE YOU A WELL-ROUNDED PERSON?

Question: So, tell us a little about yourself.

In other words: Why are you here?

Answer: Dig out those worksheets and compile a brief summary of your accomplishments. In 250 words or less, cover the following points:

1. Your strongest skills
2. Specific areas of knowledge
3. Greatest personality strengths
4. What you do best
5. Key accomplishments

(Note: All of your answers do not have to be medically oriented.)

Question: You have had several jobs in the past; how do we know you will finish the program if we accept you?

In other words: Do you have commitment and staying power?

Answer: This should be a two-part answer:

1. Admit to having moved around a bit. (It's obvious from your application.)
2. Convince the committee that you've "seen the light," if you will, and tell them what specific steps you've taken to achieve your goal.

Question: Why do you think Duke turned you down?

In other words: Did you take the time to find out why they didn't accept you?

Answer: If you interviewed elsewhere, or if you've been turned down for any reason, be sure to follow up on how you can improve your application. The program will usually tell you why you came up short this time.

"I was told that although I was a good applicant, the pool was so competitive this year that not all good candidates could feasibly be accepted. They told me to continue with my current medical experience."

Question: What are your strengths as an applicant?

In other words: Convince us that you are our woman/man.

Answer: We've already answered a similar question above. Be sure to toot your own horn without being too cocky. Review your worksheets for all of the information you'll need on this one.

Question: What are your biggest weaknesses as an applicant, and what do you plan to do to correct them?

In other words: Please tell us that you don't "walk on water" too.

Answer: They may be handing you a rope here, but you don't have to hang yourself. Everyone has weaknesses, but for an interview, you want to stay focused on the positive. Achieve a compromise: "I tend to work too many hours lately, but I realize how important my free time is and I'm much happier when I get to do the things I love outside of work."

Question: Do you manage your time well?

In other words: Can you handle a program as difficult as this? Will you require constant help?

Answer: "Yes, I do. I have a set of written goals, and I prioritize my time so as to accomplish them all in the order of their importance, and in a timely manner." (I told you having written goals is important.)

THEY MAY BE HANDING YOU A ROPE HERE, BUT YOU DON'T HAVE TO HANG YOURSELF.

Question: Do you prefer to work with others or by yourself?

In other words: How do you get along with your co-workers?

Answer: "I get along very well with others. I usually reach out to people, or I can simply hold your hand and be a friend in time of need. I consider myself to be a team player."

Question: Your supervising MD tells you to do something that you know is dead wrong; what do you do?

In other words: How's your judgment?

Answer: "I certainly do not know what it is like to be a PA in that situation, but it seems that I would have to bring the possible error to his/her attention, tactfully, and be sure that it gets resolved." A little humility goes a long way.

Question: What interests you most about our school?

In other words: Have you done your homework?

Answer: This is a very personal choice; just be prepared for the question and answer it to the best of your ability. Let the committee know that you have specific reasons for being interested in their school.

Question: What would be your ideal job as a PA?

In other words: Are you open-minded?

Answer: The key here is to show that you have an open mind, yet don't try to deceive the committee. If all of your experience is in orthopedics, don't try to tell the committee that you've always wanted to work in an HIV clinic. Give a well-balanced answer.

"Although I feel my current interest is in orthopedics, I have never worked in any other area. I know from talking with several of your graduate students that they came into the program with certain inclinations; but after doing a rotation in another specialty, they liked it enough to work in that area after graduation. I will try to keep an open mind."

Question: What did you learn from your overseas internship/experience?

In other words: What did you learn from your overseas internship/experience?

Answer: That's right, this question is as straightforward as they come, yet too many applicants blow it. Think about your travel overseas, and be prepared to discuss the impact it had on you. Did you take advantage of the local culture? Did you mix with the natives? Did you make any lasting friendships? You didn't blow this opportunity, did you?

Question: What do you want to be doing five years from now?

In other words: Do you have any goals?

Answer: Of course, you do. I won't comment much more here other than to say that I hope you still want to be a PA in five years, and that you still want to contribute to the medical community in a positive way. (Note: If you haven't filled out your goal sheet yet, please do so now.)

Question: Have you ever seen anyone die?

In other words: Are you prepared to deal with death?

Answer: This was a favorite question of one of our committee members, usually before the applicant sat down. If you have never seen anyone die, that's okay. You are not expected to know what it is like to be a PA. If you have seen someone die, reflect on the situation with empathy and explain that you are capable of carrying on. *Death is a part of life.* Don't answer, as one applicant did, "Of course, I've seen people die. I was in a gang."

Innocent Questions?

THERE ARE NO INNOCENT QUESTIONS.

There are no innocent questions. Remember, you are being evaluated from the time you walk into the building until the time you get into your car.

Question: How are you today?

In other words: Are you a positive or negative person?

Answer: "I'm fine, thank you." That's all that is required. Do not go on about the parking lot being full, or the terrible night's sleep you had, or how nervous you are.

Question: Did you have any trouble finding us?

In other words: Did you use the resources available to you?

Answer: "No trouble at all; I called the office ahead of time and got great directions from Betty."

Question: What was the last movie you saw?

In other words: What are you interested in?

Answer: I can't tell you what kind of movies to go see. Personally, your author is into horror movies, but I wouldn't tell the admission's committee that. An Oscar winner is always a safe bet.

Question: What was the most difficult question they asked you at Bowman Gray?

In other words: Have you thought about that interview?

Answer: For some reason this question draws the most tears out of applicants. One applicant said, "My mother." She was obviously emotionally distraught. Try not to get too emotional at the interview; the committee may take this as being a sign of weakness. Tell the committee that you were well prepared for the interview, and they did not ask you any questions that you did not anticipate.

CLOSING THE INTERVIEW

Question: What will you do if you don't get in this year?

In other words: Will you give up?

Answer: In Appendix A I cover specific steps to take if you do not get in this year. Do not read too much into this question. They ask this of everyone and want to know if you will apply again.

"I will consult with the program director, find out why I was not accepted, and strive to accomplish those things for next year."

Question: Do you have any questions for us? (We discuss this question and the answer to it in the previous chapter.)

Finally, it is worth repeating that you should not use these same answers at the interview. Study your worksheets and spend some time compiling your own answers to these questions. Be honest and genuine. Remember, what's the worst thing that can happen?

Financial Aid

THE ALL-IMPORTANT QUESTION

Can I afford to go to PA school? The question you should be asking is, Can I afford not to go to PA school? If your goal is to become a PA, then the answer to this question is easy. The worst thing you can do is shy away from applying because you think you won't be able to afford it, and then live the rest of your life wondering, *What if?*

When I applied to Yale and spoke to students at the open house, they told me that if I got accepted the program would do its best to ensure I got through financially. They were right. I may have borrowed a little more than I intended, but the money was available. As you will soon find out, there are plenty of opportunities for loans, grants, scholarships, etc. It does, however, take a little work on your part. But since you have set your goals and you're focused, you are prepared for anything.

The following chapter is not meant to be a step-by-step guide for filling out financial aid forms. The focus of this book, remember, is getting into the PA school of your choice. The purpose of this chapter is to give you some valuable resources and advice on getting financial aid.

THE PLAN OF ACTION

I can still remember the butterflies I felt in my stomach when I sent my deposit in to Yale. Reality set in: *I'm going to PA school.* Immediately, the thoughts began racing in my head: *I'm giving up my annual salary, plus I'm paying close to $14,000 per year for tuition, plus I'm borrowing money for living expenses and to support my family.* I began doing the math and doubt started to slowly creep in. However, I quickly remembered my goals and how hard I had worked to get this far. I needed to stay the course and get focused.

I knew somehow that everything would work out for the best. I don't regret one minute of my decision. In fact, I'm happier than I ever thought I would be. I also fully recovered from the financial strain. Here's how:

Budget

We've all heard this word before and have probably tried to write down our *income* on one side of a piece of paper and our *expenses* on the other. The problem is that we usually have a lot more expenses than we're willing

CAN I AFFORD NOT TO GO TO PA SCHOOL?

to write down. The only effective way to properly attempt a budget is to write down every penny you spend for at least one month. Everything counts, from dinner to clothes to a can of Coke. If you're married, your spouse will have to participate too. After 30 days, count up how much you spend and compare it to your original calculations. I think you'll be shocked at how much more you actually spend. But don't worry; now you can realistically see where all of your money is going and figure out ways to cut the fat.

To prepare you for some of the expenses that you'll encounter when attending PA school, I've included a list of items that you'll most likely have to spend money on:

- ▶ Rent/Mortgage
- ▶ Groceries
- ▶ Utilities
- ▶ Telephone
- ▶ Clothes
- ▶ Laundry/Dry Cleaning
- ▶ Entertainment
- ▶ Personal Expenses
- ▶ Transportation
- ▶ Books
- ▶ Other
- ▶ Travel
- ▶ Insurance
- ▶ Medical
- ▶ Medical Equipment (stethoscope, otoscope, etc.)
- ▶ Child Care
- ▶ Credit Cards
- ▶ Tuition
- ▶ Fees
- ▶ Parking
- ▶ Miscellaneous

Explore Your Options

The biggest mistake I made in PA school, now that I look back on it, was quitting my part-time job. Every program will tell you that you can't work while in PA school. You get so worked up about finally getting accepted that you absolutely want to do your best. You think that by not working you will be able to concentrate more on school. The problem is, if you're flat broke at the end of the semester, and your next financial aid check is still weeks away, you won't be able to concentrate too well anyway. You might as well work. I gave up a part-time job that paid about $300 per week. Do some quick math and you'll see that's over $15,000 per year. Ouch!

On the other hand, if you really don't need the money, then definitely don't work. It will be especially hard to keep a job once you start clinical rotations. This is definitely a personal choice. All I'm trying to tell you is to use your own judgment; every program will advise you against working, but, ultimately you have to make the decision that's best for you.

NEED-BASED AID

You will hear the term *need-based* aid a lot once you begin filling out the vast number of financial aid forms. Need-based aid is available to help you finance your PA education. Since you and your family are expected to contribute to the cost of this education, this aid is supplementary.

Need Formula

Cost of attendance (−) Student Contribution = Student Financial Need

As I mentioned already, once I got accepted to Yale, they assured me that I would have every opportunity to complete the program, regardless of my ability to pay. This, in fact, is the underlying philosophy of need-based aid:

- ▶ Access: To a program that best suits your needs
- ▶ Persistence: Inability to pay should not prevent you from finishing school
- ▶ Fairness: Your family contribution will be determined fairly.

Who Is an Independent Student?

Until July 23, 1992, all graduate students were considered independent, for federal aid purposes, if they were over 24 years old, or under 24 and not claimed as a dependent on anyone's income tax statement for the first calendar year in which they were seeking aid.

However, most schools ask for parental information even if you are totally independent and left the nest 20 years ago. You will be asked to obtain your parents' tax returns and pertinent financial information.

I personally did not ask my mom for her information, and since I did not submit any of her financial records, I left myself at risk for not receiving certain funds. In other words, if there was money left over after all other students who did submit parental information were taken care of, then I could receive that same aid.

HOW IS NEED DETERMINED?

Most PA programs should provide you with a budget worksheet that you can use to determine your cost of attendance for that institution. Below is a sample worksheet.

Need Analysis

Your financial contribution is based on a congressional formula called Congressional Methodology (CM). Need analysis is a process used to estimate how much you will need to supplement your theoretically available resources. The two components include cost of attendance and an estimate of your family's ability to contribute.

> **Congressional Methodology (CM):** CM uses taxable and nontaxable base-year income to calculate the expected student contribution (SC).
>
> **Student Contribution (SC):** This is the amount you and your spouse are expected to contribute to finance your education. This amount is the same for all schools. Once this figure is determined, it is subtracted from the cost of attendance, and the remaining amount is your financial need.
>
> The resources used to calculate the SC include items like savings, school year earnings, and spousal income. Your expected contribution is based on an analysis of your income and asset information, size of household, and number of family members in college.
>
> Students are expected to contribute 35% of their assets each year to meet educational needs.
>
> **Parental Contribution (PC):** This includes calculations based on parental income, expenses, and assets. Income includes items like social security, welfare, and dividends, as well as job salaries.

Professional Judgment

About now you may be asking, "Does anyone, besides a computer, ever look at my financial information and make a personal decision based on my cir-

STUDENTS ARE EXPECTED TO CONTRIBUTE 35% OF THEIR ASSETS EACH YEAR TO MEET EDUCATIONAL NEEDS.

cumstances?" The answer is yes. The financial aid counselor knows that even though you made $30,000 last year, you will lose some or all of that income this year. The counselor will use his professional judgment when allowing or disallowing certain funds. Needless to say, make friends with someone in the financial aid office quickly.

ORGANIZE YOUR FINANCIAL RECORDS

Suggestions

1. Follow instructions on every form.
2. Copy all forms.
3. Keep separate folders for each school.
4. Keep copies of at least two years' tax returns.
5. Gather all account numbers on bank statements, stocks, mutual funds, etc.
6. Obtain all signatures from parents, spouse, etc.
7. Put your name and social security number on all pages.
8. Respond immediately to all requests from lenders.
9. Follow up on everything.
10. Report any change in status immediately.

FEDERAL FINANCIAL AID (TITLE IV & TITLE IX)

Title IV

As part of the Higher Education Act, to qualify for this federal money you must meet the following requirements:

1. Be enrolled as a student in a specific program.
2. Be a U.S. citizen or eligible noncitizen.
3. Be making satisfactory progress in your course of study.
4. Neither be in default nor owe a refund for any federal aid received in the past.
5. Be enrolled at least half-time (6 semester hours).

Address questions to:

▶ Federal Student Aid Information Center Hotline (1-800-333-INFO)
▶ (301) 369-0518 is the TDD number for the hearing impaired.

Use this number to check and explain which schools participate, eligibility requirements, how awards are determined, complaints, the verification process, and to order publications.

Title IX

The purpose of these programs is to encourage and support graduate and professional programs in providing incentives and support for U.S. citizens, especially women and under-represented groups, to complete master's and doctoral programs. These programs are divided into six parts, A–G, although only parts A–C apply to PA programs.

Part A: Grants to institutions and consortia to encourage women and minority participation in graduate education. These grants are made to schools to help them identify talented **undergraduates** who demonstrate financial need.

Part B: Patricia Roberts Harris Fellowship Program. Provided to schools to distribute among master's, doctoral, and professional students. Distributed as follows to **minority students and women:**

- ▶ 50% master's and professional study
- ▶ 50% fellowship for doctoral study

Part C: Jacob Javits Fellowship. Available for graduate students studying in the arts, humanities, and social sciences.

Contact: Ms. Diana Haymond, Director
Jacob Javits Fellowship Program
U.S. Department of Education
400 Maryland Avenue, SW, ROB-3
Washington, DC 20202-5251
202-708-9415

OTHER FEDERAL GRANT PROGRAMS

Department of Health and Human Services (HHS), National Institutes of Health (NIH)—Public Health Service Commission Corps (COSTEP): These are service-related awards. You will be assigned to one of eight Public Health Agencies and be required to provide clinical or research services, for a monthly stipend ($1,950 for a single person). Deadlines for the COSTEP applications are December 31 for positions available May 1 through August 31; May 1 for positions September 1 through December 31; and October 1 for positions January 1 through April 30. You will be eligible to participate in this program during your clinical phase.

Contact: COSTEP
PHS Recruitment
8201 Greensboro Drive
Suite 600
McLean, VA 22102
800-221-9393

National Health Service Corps (NHSC)

An excellent program, this award covers tuition and provides you with a monthly stipend. You will incur a two-year obligation to a designated location (under-served). You will be given several sites to select from throughout the country. You will be required to make contact with these sites for availability and to negotiate a salary. Four hundred awards are given out per year. You must fill out a questionnaire and an application to be considered for an award.

Contact: NHSC Scholarships
8201 Greensboro Drive, #600
McLean, VA 22102
(800) 221-9393
In VA: (703) 734-6855

Indian Health Service (IHS)

A minimum two-year obligation for two years of financial support. Priority is given to Indian students, but others may apply.

Contact: IHS Scholarship Office at (800) 962-2817

Department of Veteran Affairs Health Professional Scholarship Program

Contact: (202) 565-7528

FEDERAL LOAN PROGRAMS

Federal Stafford Student Loan Program

These loans are offered through your bank, credit union, or other lending institutions. Graduate students may borrow up to $8,500 per year up to a total of $65,000. To qualify for a Stafford loan, you must demonstrate financial need as determined by the CM formula mentioned above.

The interest rate varies. These loans are based on need, not creditworthiness. Therefore, no cosigner is necessary.

Sample Repayment Table for Stafford Loan

If your interest rate is 8%: # months to pay in full

Loan Amount	60	72	84	96	108	120
$1,000	20.28	17.54	15.59	14.14	13.02	12.14
5,000	101.39	87.67	77.94	70.69	65.10	60.67
6,000	121.66	105.20	93.52	84.83	78.12	72.80
6,500	131.80	113.97	101.32	91.90	84.63	78.87
7,500	152.08	131.50	116.90	106.03	97.65	91.00

Source: US Department of Education

Federal Perkins Loan

This is a great loan, currently at 5% interest, available to undergraduate and graduate students. You apply for this loan, and you get the money from your individual school rather than the bank. You can borrow up to $5,000 per year for a maximum of $30,000. To qualify for this loan, you must demonstrate financial need as determined by your financial aid application. This is the loan that you may not receive if you fail to include your parents' financial information with your application.

Sample Repayment Table for Federal Perkins Loan

Total Indebtedness	Number of Payments	Monthly Payment	Total Interest Charges	Total Repaid
$4,500	120	$47.73	$1,227.60	$5,727.60
9,000	120	95.46	2,455.20	11,455.20
18,000	120	190.92	4,910.40	22,910.40

Source: US Department of Education

Federal Supplemental Loan for Students (SLS)

These loans are not as desirable as the above two programs; however, they can be a great source of money if you need more than you can get with the above programs. You obtain these loans from a commercial lender, with the interest rate being tied to the 52-week Treasury bill (T-Bill), not to exceed 11%. You may borrow up to $10,000 per year for a maximum of $73,000. The loan amount is based on your educational costs minus any other financial aid you receive.

State Programs

State programs include loan forgiveness, for which you can work at a designated clinic or site in an under-served area and receive up to $20,000 in loan forgiveness. Another good program is the Health Profession Shortage Area (HPSA) program, which provides loans at a dollar-for-dollar match for educational loans.

Contact: NHSC
Site Development and Placement Branch
4350 East-West Highway, 8th Floor
Bethesda, MD 20814
(301) 594-4165
Fax: (301) 594-4077

AAPA Constituent Chapters

Most of the state chapters of the AAPA offer some sort of scholarship program for students. Contact your state chapter for availability (Appendix E).

PA Program Tuition and Costs (Estimated)

Program	Resident	Non-Resident	Months
University of Alabama at Birmingham	$20,000	$33,000	24
University of South Alabama	$24,000		27
Arizona School of Health Sciences	$36,120	Same	24
Midwestern University	$33,424	Same	24
Charles R. Drew University of Medicine and Science	$20,000 bachelor's $18,200 certificate	Same	24
Keck School of Medicine at the University of Southern California	$79,392	?	33
Loma Linda University	$50,000	Same	23
Riverside Community College	$4,608	$16,534	24
Samuel Merritt College	$50,810	Same	28
Stanford University	$10,330	$16,630	15
Touro University Mare Island	$51,000	Same	32
University of California Davis	$11,000	$32,100	7 quarters
Western University of Health Sciences	$41,400	Same	24
Red Rocks Community College	$21,000	$30,000	24
University of Colorado Health Sciences Center	$19,160	$31,000	36
Quinnipiac University	$42,600	Same	27
Yale University	$42,900	Same	25
George Washington University PA/MPH	N/A	$70,000	37
George Washington University	N/A	$45,000	24
Howard University	$26,775	Same	24
Barry University	$42,433	Same	29
Miami-Dade Community College	$18,480	$25,074	22
Nova Southeastern University	$44,322	$46,083	27
University of Florida	$13,093	$45,666	24
Emory University	$36,603	Same	28
Medical College of Georgia	$9,204	$32,898	24
South University Bachelor's completed	$41,400	Same	27

Program	Resident	Non-Resident	Months
South University Two-years college completed	$44,055	Same	27
Idaho State University	$30,804	$42,816	24
Cook County Hospital/Malcolm X College	$4,000	$15,000	25
Finch University of Health Sciences/ Chicago Medical School	$37,194	Same	24
Midwestern University (Master's Track)	$39,193	$43,200	27
Midwestern University (Bachelor's Track)	$27,640	$30,316	24
Southern Illinois University	$20,000	$40,000	26
Butler University/Clarian Health	$43,310	Same	21
University of Saint Francis	$46,000	Same	27
Des Moines University-Osteopathic Medical Center	$36,150	Same	25
University of Iowa	$13,164	$41,316	25
Wichita State University	$7,622	$25,920	24
University of Kentucky	$15,741	$44,217	30
Louisiana State University Health Sciences Center	$8,000	$15,000	27
University of New England	$40,120	Same	24
Anne Arundel Community College	$15,025	$20,525	26
Towson University CCBC	$14,000	$28,000	26
University of Maryland Eastern Shore	$18,516	$27,484	24
Massachusetts	$48,400	Same	21
College of Pharmacy and Health Sciences	$126,400	?	57
Northeastern University	$35,870	Same	24
Springfield College/	$66,000	Same	48
Baystate Health System	$33,000		24
Central Michigan University	$30,000	$50,000	27
Grand Valley State University	$22,000	$47,300	8 semesters
University of Detroit Mercy	$41,400	Same	24–36
Wayne State University	$10,220	$22,500	24
Western Michigan University	$18,191	$43,300	24
Augsburg College	$50,050	Same	36
Saint Louis University	$49,805	Same	27
Southwest Missouri State University	$11,205	$22,410	24
Rocky Mountain College	$18,500	Same	24
Union College	$39,600	Same	27
University of Nebraska Medical Center	$16,482	$42,527	28
Manchester Center for Health Sciences of the MCPHS Graduate Program	$60,000	Same	24
Seton Hall University	$58,956	Same	36
UMDNJ and Rutgers University	$299/credit hour Maximum of 18 credits/semester	$449/credit hour Maximum of 18 credits/ semester	36

Program	Resident	Non-Resident	Months
The University of New Mexico	$10,114	$29,847	25
University of St. Francis	$45,668	Same	27
Albany-Hudson Valley	$7,050	$12,727	24
Bronx Lebanon Hospital Center	$25,000	Same	27
Brooklyn Hospital Center/ Long Island University	$24,000	Same	24
D'Youville College	$51,906	Same	42
Daemen College	$75,000 BS/MS	Same	57
Daemen College	$46,000 MS	Same	33
Hofstra University	$35,670	Same	27
LeMoyne College	$44,465	Same	24
Mercy College Graduate Program in PA Studies	$40,500	Same	27
New York Institute of Technology	$47,875	Same	28
Pace University- Lenox Hill Hospital	$43,000 24 months $82,000 48 months	Same	24–48
Rochester Institute of Technology	$78,000	Same	48
Saint Vincent Catholic Medical Centers of New York, Brooklyn & Queens Region	$26,000	Same	23
St. Vincent Catholic Medical Centers of New York, Staten Island Region	$24,000	Same	23
Stony Brook University	$11,200	$24,400	24
SUNY Downstate Medical Center	$12,392	$29,716	27
The Sophie Davis School of Biomedical Education CUNY Medical School at Harlem Hospital Center	$11,241	$23,541	31
Touro College-Bay Shore	$30,500	Same	23
Touro College-Manhattan Campus	$29,600	Same	28
Touro College-Winthrop University Hospital	$30,500	Same	23
Wagner College/Staten Island University Hospital	$38,400	Same	24
Weill Cornell Medical College	$33,884	Same	26
Duke University	$47,250	Same	25
East Carolina University	$6,992	?	24
Methodist College	$40,000 (must have bachelor's)	Same	27
Methodist College	$39,000	Same	27
Wake Forest University School of Medicine	$37,000	Same	24
University of North Dakota	To be determined	To be determined	20
Cuyahoga Community College PA Program	$4,700	$6,100	22
Cuyahoga Community College Surgical PA Program	$4,900	$6,600	22
Kettering College of Medical Arts	$40,200	Same	22

Program	Resident	Non-Resident	Months
Kettering College of Medical Arts	$47,020	Same	30
Marietta College	$49,440	Same	27
Medical College of Ohio	$19,000	$34,000	24
The University of Findlay	$41,700	Same	26
University of Oklahoma	$15,000	$45,000	30
Oregon Health & Science University	$34,749	$46,332	26
Pacific University	$45,000	Same	28
Arcadia University	$45,000	Same	24
Chatham College	$53,000	Same	24
DeSales University	$96,000	Same	36
Drexel University	$47,110	Same	27
Duquesne University	$52,632	Same	27
Gannon University	$38,000	Same	24
Gannon University	$80,000 (60-month entry-level)	Same	60
King's College	$60,750 (master's)	Same	24
King's College	$43,360 (certificate)	Same	24
Lock Haven University	$20,477	$32,056	24
Marywood University	$40,000	Same	24
Pennsylvania College of Technology	$26,500	$32,500	24
Philadelphia College of Osteopathic Medicine	$35,000	Same	24
Philadelphia University	$42,000 MS $88,236 BS/MS	Same	25 5-year program
Saint Francis University	$93,366	Same	60
Saint Francis University	$46,436	Same	24
Seton Hall University	$30,450 (pre-professional phase) $46,500 (professional phase)	Same	27
Medical University of South Carolina	$22,000	$63,000	27
University of South Dakota	$7,540	$23,972	24
Bethel College	$33,000	Same	24
Trevecca Nazarene University	$48,720	Same	27
Interservice Physician Assistant Program	N/A	N/A	24
Baylor College of Medicine	$27,000	Same	30
Texas Tech University	$5,500	$35,500	31
The University of Texas Health Science Center at San Antonio	$10,540	$31,124	36
University of North Texas Health Science Center	$6,160	$37,730	34
University of Texas Medical Branch	$5,000	$26,000	24
University of Texas Pan American	$7,166	$25,284	24
University of Texas Southwestern Medical Center	$7,550	$32,450	31
University of Utah	$24,000	$36,000	24

Program	Resident	Non-Resident	Months
College of Health Sciences	$36,300	Same	24
Eastern Virginia Medical School	$41,804	Same	27
James Madison University	$9,750	$28,400	24
Shenandoah University	$41,000	Same	27
University of Washington MEDEX	$27,213	Same	8 quarters
Alderson-Broaddus College	$54,445	Same	32
Mountain State University	$39,000	Same	34
Marquette University	$59,500	Same	32
The University of Wisconsin-LaCrosse-Gundersen Lutheran Medical Foundation-Mayo School of Health Sciences	?	?	28
University of Wisconsin-Madison	$13,000	$14,000	24

The Internet for PA School Applicants

11

The Internet is a valuable resource for the physician assistant school applicant who wants to research a particular PA program, who wants to gain more knowledge about the profession in general, or who, perhaps, wants to communicate with PAs and PA students on-line. In this chapter, I provide you with a number of web sites that should prove to be valuable to you as an applicant.

Practically every PA program in the U.S. has a web site that posts a variety of information relative to the following: admission requirements, curriculum, student societies, tuition, financial aid, and student contacts. In addition, most PA program web sites allow the user to download a program brochure and application, and to contact students who are currently attending the program.

The World Wide Web also provides a variety of organizational and personal web sites relative to the PA profession. Applicants can access these sites to learn more about current events facing the PA profession, and much more.

Internet Sites for Physician Assistant School Applicants

Source	Contribution
www.ajrassociates.com *Getting Into the PA School of Your Choice* (The author's web site)	A comprehensive and interactive site that allows applicants to ask questions of the author, sign up for one-on-one coaching with the author, join a discussion group, sign up for a free e-newsletter, link to PA programs and various PA organizations, learn about financial aid, and access FAQs.
www.aapa.org/ American Academy of Physician Assistants (AAPA)	A national organization representing physician assistants in all specialties and employment settings. Offers information for PAs, PA students, and PA wannabes.
www.saaapa.aapa.org/home.htm Student Academy of the American Academy of Physician Assistants (SAAAPA)	An information resource for physician assistant students and those interested in the PA profession.
www.apap.org/ Association of Physician Assistant Programs (APAP)	A national organization representing physician assistant programs in the U.S.
www.jaapa.com/be_core/j/index.jsp Journal of the American Academy of Physician Assistants (JAAPA)	The official journal of the American Academy of Physician Assistants (AAPA).
www.caspaonline.org Central Application Service for Physician Assistants (CASPA)	A centralized application service for applicants applying to more than one PA program.
www.ed.gov/offices/OSFAP/Students/ Federal Student (Financial) Aid	The largest source of federal student (financial) aid in the U.S.

My personal website—**www.ajrassociates.com** (***Getting Into the Physician Assistant School of Your Choice***)—is exclusively designed for the PA school applicant and provides a variety of information relative to becoming a formidable candidate for PA school. Highlights of my site include:

- ▶ *PA Links*. Find links to all of the above websites.
- ▶ *Discussion Group*. Join a PA school applicant discussion group. Learn from the experiences of other applicants who may have been through the application and interview process before.
- ▶ *Frequently Asked Questions*. Learn the answer to most of your questions relative to applying to PA school and the PA profession in general.
- ▶ *PA Programs*. A complete listing of 136 PA programs, with links to their websites.
- ▶ *About Our Book*. Find out more about my book and purchase it online if you desire.
- ▶ *Ask the Author*. A forum in which the browser can ask me questions directly via my e-mail. I personally respond to all inquiries.
- ▶ *One-on-one Coaching*. A personalized coaching service that allows the applicant to work exclusively with me on the application, essay, and interview.
- ▶ *Free e-Newsletter*. Sign up for a free monthly e-newsletter that is emailed directly to you.
- ▶ *Financial Aid*. Find out the latest news relevant to financial aid, with links to various websites.
- ▶ *Essay Tip of the Month*. Each month I place a new tip for making your essay strong and persuasive.

OTHER WEBSITES

www.aapa.org/ (American Academy of Physician Assistants)

The American Academy of Physician Assistants (AAPA) is the only national organization that represents physician assistants in all specialties and employment settings. Membership includes physician assistants, physician assistant students, physician assistant hopefuls, and those interested in supporting the physician assistant profession. The AAPA website provides volumes of information. The following is a listing of resources available on the AAPA's web site:

AAPA Information	**PA Organizations**	**About PAs**
Member Benefits and Services	**CME and Clinical Issues**	**Government Issues**
Reimbursement Issues	**Professional Practice Issues**	**Employment and Employer's Guide**
Support the PA Profession		

www.saaapa.aapa.org/home.htm (Student Academy of the American Academy of Physician Assistants)

This site provides information for current PA students but can also be a valuable resource for the PA school applicant. The applicant can use this resource to locate PA students in his/her area and to learn about the various scholarships available to PA students.

www.apap.org/ (Association of Physician Assistant Programs)

The Association of Physician Assistant Programs is the national organization representing physician assistant educational programs in the United States. APAP's mission is to assist PA educational programs in the instruction of highly educated physician assistants. The association offers an array of services for PA programs, faculty, students, and the general public, aimed at fulfilling this mission.

Prospective PA students can subscribe to the on-line *PA Programs Directory* while visiting APAP's web site. The directory is a complete listing of all of the PA programs in the U.S., including information on tuition, prerequisites, curriculum, length of training, financial aid, class size, and application deadlines.

www.jaapa.com/be core/j/index.jsp (Official Journal of the American Academy of Physician Assistants)

This is the official journal of the AAPA and is clinically oriented, geared toward practicing PAs and PA students. In addition to clinical articles, the journal frequently reports on issues relevant to the PA profession. The journal also provides a listing of employment opportunities.

www.caspaonline.org (Central Application Service for Physician Assistants)

The Central Application Service for Physician Assistants (CASPA) offers a web-based application service that allows PA school applicants to apply to numerous participating educational programs by completing a single application.

www.ed.gov/offices/OSFAP/Students/ (Federal Student Aid)

The Federal Student Aid Homepage provides information relative to financial aid available from the U.S. Department of Education. The Federal Student Aid programs are the largest source of student aid in America, providing over $60 billion a year in grants, loans, and work-study assistance. Here you'll find help for every stage of the financial aid process, whether you're in school or out of school.

PA FORUMS ON THE INTERNET

This last section covers a listing of PA forums available on the Internet. By joining a forum, an applicant can get plugged in to some of the hot topics facing the profession and get a sense for what PAs in general are thinking. The applicant can also pose questions to the forum and perhaps locate PAs to shadow. There are five listservs to provide a variety of forums for PAs and those interested in the PA profession. Subscriptions are free, but you must be a subscriber to post to the forums. Once the server acknowledges your subscription(s) you may post to the list(s).

PA Professional Forum: PAs discussing general interest and nonclinical topics. Subscribe via the Web at http://list.mc.duke.edu/archives/paforum.html; post messages to paforum@list.mc.duke.edu

Primary Care PA Forum: PAs discuss clinical topics. Subscribe via the Web at http://list.mc.duke.edu/archives/primarypa.html; post messages to primarypa@list.mc.duke.edu

Student PA Forum: Communicate with fellow students and prospective students. Subscribe via the Web at http://list.mc.duke.edu/archives/studentpa.html; post messages to studentpa@list.mc.duke.edu

PA Faculty Forum: Exchange ideas with PA program faculty. Subscribe via the Web at http://list.mc.duke.edu/archives/pafaculty.html; post messages to pafaculty@list.mc.duke.edu

Physician Assistant Journal: See articles and reviews of PA literature as well as Continuing Medical Education (CME) offerings and potential jobs. Subscribe via the Web at http://list.mc.duke.edu/archives/pajournal.html; post messages to pajournal@list.mc.duke.edu

The Internet is a valuable resource for PA school applicants. The applicant can learn volumes about the PA profession by visiting some of these key sites. In addition, it is possible to develop a rapport with PAs and PA students who may become mentors to you and who may also provide you with shadowing opportunities. Good luck with your search!

PA Job Descriptions

12

This chapter is designed to introduce the PA school applicant to the various clinical specialties and disciplines in which PAs practice. I will cover the seven areas of clinical medicine (family practice, emergency medicine, pediatrics, psychiatry, obstetrics and gynecology (Ob-Gyn), internal medicine, and surgery) that many programs require as mandatory rotations.

Each of the above specialties will be described as follows:

1. *Description of Duties*
2. *The Team*
3. *Salary*
4. *Summary*

The *Description of Duties* is an account of the day-to-day activities and functions of a PA working in a given specialty. I will point out the various clinical presentations and types of patients you can expect to evaluate and treat in that particular discipline, and try to give you a sense of the physical and mental challenges associated with the job. For instance, some areas of medicine are more cerebral than others, while other specialties tend to be more task- and procedure-oriented.

After reading over the various job descriptions, the reader may come to some insightful conclusions. For instance, you may be surprised to find out that the traditional family practice PA doesn't necessarily get to spend a great deal of time with his or her patients, as reported in most of the PA literature. Many family practice PAs are so busy that they barely have time for lunch. You may be surprised to find out that the surgery PA actually has more of an opportunity to get to know the patient, and the patient's family, much better since he or she may have that patient on his/her service for several days.

I bring up this point because the premise of this book is to set you apart from the competition. Many applicants come to the interview without a clue as to how real PAs function. They think we have unlimited time to spend with our patients. It's refreshing, and it shows a great deal of insight, when an applicant is knowledgeable about the different jobs we perform and understands that what the literature says and what PAs actually do may be two different things.

During the course of interviews, 90% of applicants will say that they want to work in family practice or with AIDS patients. They think this is

YOU MAY BE SURPRISED TO FIND OUT THAT THE TRADITIONAL FAMILY PRACTICE PA DOESN'T NECESSARILY GET TO SPEND A GREAT DEAL OF TIME WITH HIS OR HER PATIENTS, AS REPORTED IN MOST OF THE PA LITERATURE.

the politically correct answer. They fail to realize, however, that the people interviewing them are real PAs working in a variety of specialties. Less than 40% of all PAs work in family practice; that leaves more than 60% of all PAs to work in other areas. We need PAs in every specialty. I can't tell you how many applicants will come to the interview with, for example, six years of orthopedic experience and then tell you that they want to work in an AIDS clinic. That may be a legitimate goal for some, but most are not being true to the committee, or themselves. The key is to be consistent and to be honest. Don't fake it, because it won't work!

The Team consists of the professionals you will interact with the most on a daily basis. Our profession is one in which we must work in collaboration with a variety of medical, and nonmedical, personnel. The closer you keep the "team concept" to your understanding of our profession the better off you'll be at interview time.

The *Salary* is self-explanatory. I simply try to give you an idea of the earning potential of PAs in a variety of settings. Of course, these numbers will vary depending on the type of practice (hospital versus clinic versus private practice) and your negotiating skills.

The *Summary* is a quick and concise synopsis of the stress level, hours, educational opportunities, research opportunities, and pace of the job. The summary also gives you an overall "gestalt" for which type of person generally gravitates toward each specialty.

FAMILY PRACTICE

Description of Duties. This area is the cornerstone of our profession; approximately 40% of all PAs work in family practice. The family practice PA may work in a clinic (urban or rural) or for a private physician or group of physicians. PAs working in family practice generally require a strong breadth of knowledge in the following areas: pediatrics, internal medicine, dermatology, orthopedics, HIV, cardiology, endocrinology, pulmonology, obstetrics and gynecology, and renal disease. In addition, he/she must develop the skills to perform minor surgery, splint and cast limbs, and remove foreign bodies from eyes, to name just a few.

The patients seen in a family practice setting are generally nonacute, except, perhaps, in a rural setting where your practice may be the only medical provider for miles. Many of the patients are familiar to the practice and typically present with colds, flu, and minor ailments. Others, however, may present with more complex problems and require closer follow-up. Depending on the type and location of the practice, you may follow a great number of HIV and AIDS patients. You may also be required to go out into the community and provide care to the indigent population. In fact, many inner city clinics cater specifically to this population.

In addition to the various acute illnesses evaluated and treated on a daily basis, there is also a very routine aspect to this job. For instance, the family practice PA performs numerous school, sports, and well-baby physical examinations. Many patients in the practice are diabetic and/or hypertensive and require periodic, routine follow-up examinations. Administering immunizations is also an important part of this job.

Of course, like all specialties, the family practice PA works very closely with his/her supervising physician(s). Although the PA works fairly autonomously in this setting, the physician is always available for consultation on the more difficult cases.

Most family practice clinics have pharmacy, x-ray, and laboratory capabilities. Depending on the size and budget of the facility, the PA may be required to perform basic laboratory studies to confirm or rule out a diagnosis.

Contrary to popular belief (of many PA school applicants), a PA working in a family practice setting doesn't always have vast amounts of time to spend with his or her patients. In fact, many PAs in a busy family practice setting will see over 40 patients per day, often skipping lunch to stay on schedule. Generally, however, the hours are fairly regular, nine to five, and there typically is no call or weekend duty.

The Team. The family practice team varies from office to office depending on the size of the practice. In general, PAs work alongside physicians, nurses, nurse practitioners, medical assistants, and various clerical personnel. A larger practice may also employ x-ray technicians, laboratory technicians, and pharmacists.

Salary. Depending on the type of practice (solo, group, hospital clinic), family practice PAs probably earn in the middle of the salary range, from $60,000 to $75,000 per year. Of course, salary is dependent on the amount of clinical experience the clinician brings to the bargaining table. Some clinics are open during the evening hours and on weekends, which provides an opportunity for the family practice PA to earn an extra $3,000 to $10,000 per year in differential pay.

Summary. The family practice setting represents a traditional role for PAs. This setting provides a great opportunity for the PA to enhance his/her clinical skills by evaluating and treating a variety of medical presentations. Although the job is not as leisurely paced as one may expect, the stress level is usually very manageable, as the patients tend to be nonacute. The job has the potential to become routine at times, but certainly not boring.

EMERGENCY MEDICINE

Description of Duties. About 8% of physician assistants work in this exciting arena. Generally, an emergency room (ER) is divided into several sections: surgery, medicine, trauma, major medical, fast track, pediatrics, and psychiatry. Some PAs will work in primarily one area, but many rotate through them all depending on preference, experience, and hospital policy.

In the surgery section, the patients usually have obvious complaints and injuries, and the PA's role is highly procedure-oriented; he/she does a lot of suturing, splinting/casting, removing foreign bodies from eyes, and wrapping sprains and strains. However, some patients may have more insidious complaints, such as appendicitis, bowel obstruction and kidney/gallstones, which involve further diagnostic work-up with x-rays and laboratory testing.

In the medicine section, the PA sees a variety of common and complex patients with complaints of asthma, fever, shortness of breath, nausea/vomiting, dizziness, etc. Many of the patients are elderly and have a history of diabetes or heart disease. The PA usually works very closely with the patient's family physician, especially when the patient has a complicated past medical history. This area of the ER is less task/procedure-oriented, and the PA is

MANY PAs IN A BUSY FAMILY PRACTICE SETTING WILL SEE OVER 40 PATIENTS PER DAY, OFTEN SKIPPING LUNCH TO STAY ON SCHEDULE.

ABOUT 8% OF PHYSICIAN ASSISTANTS WORK IN THIS EXCITING ARENA.

challenged to collect a thorough medical history and utilize excellent clinical skills to arrive at a diagnosis.

The trauma section of the ER is reserved for acute injuries sustained from motor vehicle accidents, gunshot wounds, falls, knife wounds, fights, ruptured aneurysms, and burns, to name a few. In this arena the PA will have a specific task as a member of the trauma team. Usually, a surgeon will head the team, and the PA will perform duties such as collecting blood gases, putting in a chest tube, holding pressure on an arterial bleeder, and helping insert a central line. Not all PAs who work in the ER are directly involved with the trauma team. In fact, many hospitals require additional training for the PA who wants to work in this area.

Major medicine is an area in which patients in need of acute medical attention are treated. Usually heart attack victims and patients in acute respiratory distress or cardiac arrest are triaged to this area. The PA may be the initial provider on the scene and will be responsible to initiate treatment until the attending physician arrives.

Fast track is an area designated for follow-up visits and routine, minor illnesses like sore throats, coughs, hangnails, etc. This is usually staffed by a designated PA on a daily basis, or by several PAs who rotate through on different days.

The pediatric section of the ER is usually covered by the pediatric residents, interns, or PAs. The patient's ages range from newborn babies to teenagers. Common presentations include asthma attacks, sore throats, ear infections, and fevers. Obviously, the clinicians work closely with the patient's pediatrician when forming a treatment plan. Usually, the surgical residents will handle the lacerations and broken bones.

Most ERs also have a psychiatric room/section for patients with acute psychiatric problems. In addition, the same area is generally used for intoxicated patients or highly uncooperative/combative patients. The PA has a limited role in this area, except to contact psychiatry and have the patient evaluated. The PA may have to treat lacerations, bruises, or acute overdoses prior to the psychiatric evaluation.

The Team. The team in the ER consists of a variety of clinicians, technicians, nurses, clerical personnel, security, and personnel from various emergency medical services. PAs work very closely with the attending physicians, Housestaff, consulting physicians, nurses, and technicians to ensure the best treatment for the patient.

Salary. ER PAs tend to be at the higher end of the pay scale, in part due to the stress of the job, but also due to the number of hours and various shifts worked. The range is from $60,000 to $80,000 per year.

Summary. The ER PA must be able to work in a stressful environment in collaboration with a variety of team members. The job is fast-paced, and calls for a clinician who has both excellent surgical skills and a thorough medical knowledge. Although there is usually a lot of back up available, due to the usually high patient volume, many ER PAs work autonomously, requiring little supervision.

PEDIATRICS

Description of Duties. Pediatric PAs comprise about 3% of the PA population, and either work in clinics, private pediatrician offices, or in a hospital

PA JOB DESCRIPTIONS

setting. In this section we will cover the Pediatric/Neonatal Physician Assistant in the hospital setting, i.e., the Housestaff.

The Pediatric/Neonatal PA functioning as Housestaff implies, by its very name, duties divided into and covering several areas and specialties. You are required to see patients on the in-patient pediatric floor, attend and assist with high-risk deliveries, evaluate and manage newborns (from 30 weeks' gestation on up), work in the pediatric clinic, and provide coverage to the emergency room as needed.

Usually, the job requires in-house calls and rotating shifts, as well as night and weekend coverage. As Housestaff, you may be the only clinician available for emergencies in the middle of the night. Although the attending physician is always available by phone, you will often be the first clinician on the scene to evaluate and stabilize the patient.

In pediatrics, the patients are usually admitted through the emergency room or directly from a physician's office. Your duties upon admission include performing a history and physical examination, ordering necessary tests, forming a diagnosis and treatment plan, and consulting with the attending pediatrician. You may also be required to draw blood samples, catheterize patients, and perform lumbar punctures. You then follow the patient on a daily basis, writing progress notes and discussing further diagnostic and treatment modalities with the attending pediatrician.

In neonatology, the PA medically manages newborns from 30 weeks gestation until term. The supervising physician in this area is a neonatologist. Again, as Housestaff, your responsibility is to manage the day-to-day medical care of these neonates who have a variety of acute and chronic problems. This service is very procedure-oriented, with plenty of intravenous starts, lumbar punctures, central (intravenous) line placements, ventilator management, collecting blood gases, placing chest tubes, and much more.

Attending high-risk deliveries is also a part of neonatology. Here, you are responsible for resuscitation of the newborn in the delivery room. Many times you work autonomously, with only you and the nursing staff available to revive the infant until the anesthesiologist and pediatrician arrive.

The pediatric clinic is usually reserved for scheduled, nonemergent patients. This is where the PA performs well-baby check-ups, gives immunizations, and sees a variety of colds, earaches, and sore throats. The acuity of the patients is not as high as in neonatology, but the pace can be fast and furious.

Common calls to the emergency room are for asthma attacks, broken bones, and high fevers. On occasion, however, you may see a patient suffering from cardiac arrest or an acute overdose. In addition, many families without medical insurance will bring their children to the emergency room for routine visits: colds, coughs, and rashes. Surgical injuries are usually deferred to the surgical PAs or Housestaff.

The Team. The pediatric team consists of pediatricians, neonatologists, residents, interns, physician assistants, nurses, respiratory therapists, occupational therapists, nurse's aides, unit clerks, and secretaries.

Salary. Pediatric PAs tend to be at the middle of the pay scale with respect to PAs in other specialties. The range is from $60,000 to $75,000, depending on the hours worked.

Summary. This is a job in which there is a lot of calm, followed by moments of chaos. You must be willing and able to work various shifts, including nights, weekends, and holidays. The stress level ranges from extremely high when dealing with critically ill newborns to fairly routine when working in the clinic. You need to be well organized, and, at times, ready to be in two places at one time. This is not a job for the PA lacking in confidence and maturity.

PSYCHIATRY

Description of Duties. Psychiatry PAs generally work in either a hospital-based setting or in a clinic/mental health center. Approximately 3% of all PAs work in psychiatry.

In the hospital setting, PAs will either work on a consultation service or on the psychiatric ward of the facility. On the consultation (consult) service, the PA will be called to evaluate in-patients from any area of the hospital—surgery or medicine. Working closely with the psychiatrist in this setting, the PA will evaluate patients for depression, anxiety, alcohol withdrawal, psychiatric medication problems, dementia, delirium, and, quite common to elderly Intensive Care Unit patients, "sun-downing." Many of these patients have a history of psychiatric illness and simply need to be followed while in the hospital. Others, however, may present new symptoms and may require a more detailed work-up.

Once the patient is seen and evaluated, the PA discusses the case with his/her attending or hospital-based psychiatrist and consults with the patient's attending physician as to the recommendation. Many times the recommendation is to change a medication or simply hold it for a period of time. Occasionally, the PA will recommend further testing, especially with patients who present with new findings. The PA may recommend a neurology consult or an MRI or CT scan to rule out certain pathology.

The PA will then follow all of the patients on the consult service, usually daily, writing notes and continuing recommendations until the patient is discharged or stable enough to not warrant further consultation.

PAs working in the psychiatric ward of the hospital and a clinic/mental health center have similar duties and will be covered together here. Many of these clinics treat a great deal of substance abuse patients (alcohol and drug) and patients considered to have "dual diagnosis" (substance abuse and psychiatric illness), for example, a patient suffering from alcoholism and schizophrenia. The patients may be treated on an in-patient or out-patient basis. The PA's role in this area is usually to take care of the patient's medical needs: physical examinations, monitoring the patient's non-psychiatric medications, hypertension, diabetes, seizures, etc. The PA may also be responsible for giving classes to the patients on topics such as AIDS, hepatitis, and nutrition.

Some PAs choose work in this area because of the opportunity to be involved in research. Many clinics offer experimental drugs and/or treatment programs to the patients who are struggling with alcohol or drug problems, and who have failed conventional treatment. The PA is more involved in counseling and group therapy than in the medical aspect of the treatment plan.

The Team. In a hospital setting (consult service), the PA works closely with the hospital psychiatrists, the patient's family, the nursing staff, and the patient's attending physician. In the clinic setting, the team consists of psychiatrists, psychologists, social workers, counselors, nurses, attending physicians (occasionally), technicians, and clerical personnel.

Salary. Psychiatry PAs tend to be at the low range of the pay scale. The salary range is from $60,000 to $65,000.

Summary. This position is generally one of low stress. The hospital-based consult service PA works fairly autonomously, depending on his/her supervisor, and sees a variety of patients throughout the hospital. The PA working in the psychiatric clinic usually works at a slow pace and can have a tedious job at times. This may be the perfect opportunity, however, for the PA interested in doing research and publishing papers.

OB-GYN

Description of Duties. The Ob-Gyn specialty is traditionally filled by female PAs and represents about 3% of the PA workforce. This specialty deals with both obstetrics (dealing with pregnant women during their pregnancy and childbirth) and gynecology (dealing with diseases peculiar to women, primarily those of the genital tract as well as endocrinology and reproductive physiology). In this section we will discuss the role of the hospital-based Ob-Gyn PA.

This position is one of great diversity with respect to the various practice settings. The Ob-Gyn PA may work in the hospital Ob-Gyn clinic, the operating room, the in-patient Ob-Gyn floor, the maternity ward, and, where applicable, in a community van that reaches out to the indigent population in the community.

In the Ob-Gyn clinic, the PA will see women for prenatal visits, annual Pap smears, pregnancy testing, and a variety of complaints relative to the female anatomy. The PA should be proficient in the pelvic examination. The Ob-Gyn PA should have excellent communication skills, as many of the patients are teenagers and require a great deal of counseling with respect to teen pregnancy, HIV prevention, and sexually transmitted disease prevention.

In the operating room, the PA is usually a first or second assistant to the attending Ob-Gyn physician. The majority of surgical cases include hysterectomies and laparoscopic explorations of the pelvic cavity. PAs may also have a role in assisting the attending physician in cesarean section deliveries.

The in-patient Ob-Gyn floor is generally reserved for patients recovering from surgery. The PA's role is to round on all of the patients, change dressings, check labs, write progress notes, and write orders. This function is very similar to that of the surgical PA.

The maternity ward is, of course, where most of the deliveries take place. PAs generally have a limited role on this floor. Most babies are delivered by the attending physician, or by midwifes who play a significant role in many hospitals.

Some hospitals and clinics have a community van that goes out into various neighborhoods and provides routine and prenatal care to mothers who would not ordinarily come to a facility. This may be the only medical care many of these patients ever receive. This is an excellent opportunity for the PA to reach out and make a difference in the community.

THE OB-GYN SPECIALTY IS TRADITIONALLY FILLED BY FEMALE PAs.

The Team. For obvious reasons, the Ob-Gyn field is predominantly comprised of females, except for attending physicians. In addition to PAs and MDs, the team may consist of nurse practitioners, nurse midwifes, nurses, technicians, OR personnel, and clerical personnel.

Salary. Ob-Gyn PAs tend to earn average salaries with respect to PAs in other areas. The range is from $60,000 to $75,000.

Summary. This specialty is traditionally filled by female PAs. There is a great amount of diversity in Ob-Gyn, i.e., surgery, medicine, in-patient, and clinic responsibilities. This job can be both physically and mentally challenging, requiring both excellent diagnostic skills and proficient surgical capabilities.

INTERNAL MEDICINE

Description of Duties. Approximately 8% of practicing PAs work in internal medicine. In this section we will cover the hospital-based internal medicine PA. The reader should keep in mind, however, that there are many opportunities available for PAs to work with private physicians and group practices.

The medicine PA must have, or acquire, a general understanding of all the medical subspecialties: cardiology, renal medicine, pulmonology, endocrinology, neurology, dermatology, hematology, and HIV medicine. As a result, medicine makes a great first job for the new graduate who wants to build a solid foundation for future practice.

In the hospital environment, the medicine PA is usually a part of a team with other PAs and Housestaff (residents and interns). Quite commonly, a medical student or PA student will be assigned to the service also.

The typical day usually starts early in the morning with individual rounds. Each clinician will briefly see and examine his/her patients. Next comes rounds. The chief resident will gather the team and discuss each patient on the service. This usually takes place just outside of each patient's room. If the patient is new to the service, admitted overnight, the primary provider will give a brief but thorough summary of the patient's history and physical examination, laboratory results, x-ray results, diagnosis, and treatment plan. The chief residents may then question the team, or an individual member, about issues relevant to the patient's case or presentation. This procedure is affectionately called "pimping," and it is a way to keep the entire team on its toes and makes for a great daily learning experience. Morning rounds can last from two to three hours depending on the size of the service and the mood of the chief resident.

After team rounds, the PA will generally have some time to check lab results and tests, and read notes in his/her patient's charts that may have been written by consultants or the patient's attending physician. The PA will then check any lab results or tests that may have been pending and begin to write the daily note on each patient. Included in the notes are the plan for the day and any specific orders that must be carried out as part of that treatment plan.

Throughout the day, the PA touches base with attending physicians and consulting physicians with respect to the patient's progress and treatment plan. The PA will also discuss any significant findings with the chief resident, as he/she is ultimately responsible for the service.

At some point in the day, the team will meet again for x-ray rounds. An attending radiologist usually presides over the meeting, in the Department of Radiology, and will discuss each and every x-ray, ultrasound, MRI, angiogram, or CT scan that was performed on the patients on your service that morning. This is a great learning experience and helps the clinician get better acquainted with reading and interpreting various radiological studies.

In addition to team rounds and radiology rounds, the team may also have "attending rounds." Usually, one of the attending physicians is assigned to your service for the month, and may give two or three lectures a week on various topics. This may include visiting with some patients and discussing his/her clinical findings. Again, this is an excellent and valuable learning tool.

Each clinician is usually assigned one or two new admissions per day. The PA will go to the emergency room and perform a complete history and physical exam on the patient. He/she will then order any appropriate tests (labs, x-rays, etc.), touch base with the attending physician, and write the patient's admission orders. The patient is presented and discussed with the rest of the team at morning rounds.

In addition to the daily routine described above, the medicine PA must also be proficient in various diagnostic and therapeutic procedures—obtaining blood gases, performing lumbar punctures, starting IVs, drawing blood, central line placement, and thoracentesis. Usually, the chief resident will teach these various procedures to the PA and allow him/her to accomplish them as proficiency and comfort level progress.

The Team. The internal medicine team consists of PAs, residents, interns, nurses, attending physicians, consulting physicians, technicians, aides, and clerical personnel.

Salary. The salary for internal medicine PAs tends to be on the low side; this is usually due to the excellent hours and great teaching opportunities. The range is from $60,000 to $70,000.

Summary. This specialty offers great hours and low stress. In addition, this is a good job for the new graduate because of the excellent learning opportunities available. Many PAs will stay in this position for a couple of years and then move on to private practice, or specialize in one of the subspecialties. This is definitely the perfect position for the cerebral-minded PA.

SURGERY

Description of Duties. Surgery and its related subspecialties comprise an area second only to family practice in terms of total numbers of PA positions (approximately 22%). Physician assistants function effectively in multiple clinical settings, performing in-hospital surgical tasks along with and, not infrequently, in place of residents. Many hospitals employ PAs as house officers (Housestaff) in lieu of maintaining a surgical residency teaching program comprised of MDs.

Physician assistants who wish to pursue a career in surgery should be proficient in medicine. The answer to this apparent paradox becomes clear with an examination of PA responsibilities on a typical hospital surgical service. PAs, as house officers, are responsible for the preoperative, intraop-

MANY HOSPITALS EMPLOY PAs AS HOUSE OFFICERS (HOUSESTAFF) IN LIEU OF MAINTAINING A SURGICAL RESIDENCY TEACHING PROGRAM COMPRISED OF MDS.

erative, and postoperative care of surgical patients. A given patient's preoperative state of health clearly will affect his/her intraoperative and postoperative care, as well as the overall prognosis. Timely identification of any pre-existing conditions (diabetes mellitus, pulmonary disease, coronary artery disease, peripheral vascular disease, renal disease, liver disease, or compromise in the immune system), together with appropriate preoperative intervention, are critical to a favorable outcome. Similarly, there are myriad postoperative conditions that can arise: fever, pulmonary embolus, respiratory distress, renal failure, infection, and hemorrhage. These conditions can be lessened, or prevented, by the intervention of a knowledgeable surgical PA.

The responsibilities of the surgical PA include taking the patient's history, performing the physical exam, ordering appropriate tests and x-rays, writing the admission orders, and performing a preoperative check prior to the patient's surgery. In addition, postoperatively, the PA rounds on the floor, writes notes on all of the patients, changes the treatment plan as needed, and consults with the attending physician (surgeon) on a daily basis.

Intraoperatively, the PA's duties include first and second assisting. Many surgical procedures consist of the attending surgeon and the PA doing the actual surgery, with the ancillary help of the scrub nurse, circulating nurse, technicians, and anesthesiologist. The surgical PA should have a thorough knowledge of anatomy and be technically proficient in various procedures.

In addition to assisting with major surgical procedures, the surgical PA should be able to perform a variety of minor surgical and invasive procedures. These include, but are not limited to, administering local anesthesia, surgical debridement of wounds, intramuscular injections and arthrocentesis, peripheral and central venous cannulation, chest tube placement/removal, proper immobilization of various fractured bones (as well as traction where indicated), bladder catheterization, and airway management/intubation. The surgical PA should also be able to perform and interpret electrocardiograms and be Adult Cardiac Life Support (ACLS) qualified.

The surgical PA is often called to the emergency room to evaluate and admit patients to the surgical service. The ability of the surgical PA to work in collaboration with the ER team is essential. Decisions made by the PA affect not only the patient's health, but also the efforts of the nurses, lab technicians, respiratory therapists, physical and occupational therapists, and team members from other services in the hospital.

The surgical PA is usually required to take call on a rotating basis. This usually involves spending the night in the hospital, mostly in the Surgical Intensive Care Unit, but providing care to the entire service as needed.

The Team. The surgical team consists of a variety of medical and surgical personnel. Mostly, the PA works with attending surgeons, nurses, various technicians and therapists, circulating nurses, scrub nurses, and anesthesiologists (or nurse anesthetists) in the operating room, along with medical attendings, and various interns and residents.

Salary. Surgery PAs are usually on the higher end of the pay scale. This is usually due to the acuity of the patients, the hours on call, and the ability of the attending to be reimbursed for first assistant services. The range is from $60,000 to over $100,000.

THE SURGICAL PA SHOULD HAVE A THOROUGH KNOWLEDGE OF ANATOMY AND BE TECHNICALLY PROFICIENT IN VARIOUS PROCEDURES.

THIS IS DEFINITELY NOT THE JOB FOR THE SHY AND RETIRING. THE SURGICAL PA IS GENERALLY A "TYPE A" INDIVIDUAL.

Summary. This is definitely not the job for the shy and retiring. The surgical PA is generally a "Type A" individual. In addition, he or she must have excellent written and verbal communication skills, a willingness to handle responsibility, and the ability to be a team player. He or she must also be able to pay strict attention to detail.

Appendices

GRIEVING

For those of you who have taken classes in "Death and Dying," you will be familiar with the five steps involved in the grieving process: denial, anger, bargaining, depression, and acceptance. While being rejected from PA school does not compare with losing a family member, or perhaps even with losing a pet, it can still be a devastating and discouraging experience. The trick is to move through the process and get to the acceptance phase as quickly as possible. This will allow you to begin working toward improving your application for next year.

At first, you will have a hard time believing the fact that, after all of the hard work you put into the process, you weren't accepted. You may then become angry, realizing that your best-laid plans have been shattered. Your attitude may become self-defeating. The key here is not to burn any bridges, and by no means should you call the program and try to bargain, or beg, for acceptance. This will only hurt your chances for next year. Believe me, there will be a next year and it will come sooner than you think.

You will naturally be depressed, but you will eventually come to accept the fact that you didn't get in and that the sun will still rise tomorrow. Don't take things too personally, as many excellent candidates don't get into PA school on their first try. It's mostly a matter of logistics: too many good applicants for precious few slots. Get through the grieving process and get ready to go back to work.

GATHER YOUR THOUGHTS

As I have tried to point out all through this book, only 5% of applicants get accepted each year. Is it the top 5% who get in? Hardly. No system is perfect, and some poorly qualified applicants are likely to slip through the cracks and be accepted. Many of these people will also fail along the way. This is inevitable, but some schools have a higher attrition rate than others. Take comfort in knowing you're not alone and you will get another chance.

In any case, **keep a positive attitude.** You will be a much stronger, and wiser, candidate next year. You will improve your grades, gain more experience, have a better understanding of the profession, and have more time to write a great essay.

DEVELOP A PLAN

Once you become ready to pick yourself up by the bootstraps, contact the schools that you applied to this year and ask for feedback on your application. This is a critical step, as you need to find out specifically where you are lacking as a candidate. Admissions committee members usually write down notes about your application or interview. Ask for specific areas that you need to improve on based on these comments. Generally, the comments will be relevant to experience, grades, understanding of the profession, poor essay, poor interview, or "weird behavior." The last may be hard to illicit from the program director or whoever may be giving you the feedback. Make a note of any suggestions and thank the committee for considering your application or for the interview, even though you were rejected. It is important to do this right away while the application is still fresh in their minds.

Once you accomplish the above, you are ready to return to Chapter 3 and rewrite you goals. I hope by now you realize the value of doing this. Compile a concise plan of action to strengthen your application for next year. Do you need to take any classes over? Do you need more hands-on experience? How about your narrative—is it persuasive and motivating? Think carefully about how you can present yourself in a better light next year.

IMPLEMENT THE PLAN

Just do it! After you have a complete list of goals, begin working on them in order of importance. For instance, if the program director told you that the committee is concerned with your ability to handle a rigorous science course load, enroll in some hard science classes. If you are lacking experience, go out and start volunteering in the local emergency room. As a volunteer, you are usually considered an "insider" by the hospital and you may have a good shot at a paid job if one arises. Or, better yet, take a short course to become a certified nursing assistant (CNA) and get a paid job in a hospital or clinic. Jobs usually abound in this field.

Remember, the committee will look to see what you have done to improve your application over the past year. Too many people apply over and over again, but fail to make any positive changes.

NARRATIVE STATEMENT

When you fill out your application next year, be sure to write a brand new narrative statement, and obtain fresh letters of recommendation. This is very important. Let the committee know exactly what you have done to improve and strengthen your application. Point out that you have followed their advice and took an extra class or gained more hands-on experience.

The purpose of a letter of recommendation is to provide the admissions committee with a detailed description of an applicant's abilities, rather than merely checking off a few boxes on a standard form. Too many applicants feel that as long as the letter is written by a so-called "big shot," the content is irrelevant. This is simply not true and may hinder rather than help your application.

Let's look at a sample letter of recommendation for a candidate applying to PA school. Afterward, we will dissect it and point out the three key elements that make up a great letter of reference.

Dear Ms. Dean:

Please accept this letter as a strong recommendation for John Smith's application as a student in your Physician Assistant program. I am the current Dean of the College of Health and Human Performance at Mankato State University, and John was my student for four years and my teaching assistant for two years.

As a student, John was easily in the top ten percent of his peers for four years in a row. As a teaching assistant, he was rated highest by over 122 students who have taken my classes. All students respected him and admired his presentations and leadership. He proved himself a dedicated, hard-working, and diligent young man.

John served for four years in the U.S. Navy as a corpsman, and his experience in that position would give great strength to his career as a Physician Assistant. He also spent time as an officer in the U.S. Air Force, which explains his admirable ability to pay strict attention to detail.

This young man has a social conscience, high energy, a cooperative style, and the uncanny ability to analyze complex problems in the health field in simple yet constructive context. His social graces are beyond reproach. John would make an outstanding PA. He really cares for people, and people care for him.

I strongly recommend John Smith for your Physician Assistant program.

Sincerely,

Robert R. Rockingham, P.h.D.
Dean, College of Health and Human Performance
Mankato State University

CONTENT

This letter contains the three key elements of an appropriate letter of reference:

1. Introduction and background of the writer.
2. Writer's relationship to the candidate.
3. Quantified claims rather than general statements.

The purpose of the writer's introducing him/herself in the opening paragraph is to qualify as a legitimate reference. It shows that the reference truly knows the applicant and can honestly and objectively comment on his/her academic achievements, interpersonal and organizational skills, compassion, etc.

Finally, the reference quantifies his claims. When we read applications, many people appear to as though they can "walk on water." If the writer uses "meaningful specifics" versus "wandering generalities," he/she lends more credence to the letter. Example: ". . . was rated the highest by over 122 students."

IDENTIFY CANDIDATE'S STRENGTHS

A good recommendation letter does not simply recite the obvious, i.e., "Sue has a great GPA." It's quite obvious to the committee that Sue has a 3.7 GPA; they have her transcripts.

The writer should be more creative and spend enough time on the letter to make you stand out from the crowd. The writer is usually asked to evaluate you in several areas:

1. Academic performance
2. Interpersonal skills
3. Maturity
4. Adaptability/flexibility
5. Motivation for a career as a PA

The writer may comment on all of these areas or just a couple. In the area that he/she does comment on, however, the statements should be specific and relevant to the category selected. For instance:

Academic performance: ". . . top ten percent of his peers."

Interpersonal skills: "He cares for people, and people care for him."

Maturity: "All students respected him and admired his presentations and leadership."

Adaptability/flexibility: ". . . the uncanny ability to analyze complex problems . . . in simple yet constructive terms."

WHAT ABOUT WEAKNESSES?

We all have faults; the trick here is to have the evaluator mention a minor weakness and present it as though it is actually a strength. Mentioning a weakness lends objectivity and credibility to the letter of recommendation. Example: "John's strict attention to detail, at times, appeared to keep him late in the office. However, it is for this very reason that I believe he will make an excellent clinician, and will not miss any details when it comes to taking care of his patients."

ONE FINAL TIP

The writer should keep in mind that the reader of your application may have to read a hundred others before yours. It's very important to keep the letters short, concise, specific, and personal. Be sure that the writer is recommending you for PA school and not "medical school." Also, be sure that the writer changes the name of the school with each application you send in.

Fill out the following sheet and keep a copy on your person at all times. Read this sheet every morning when you arise and every evening before you retire. By reviewing your goals daily, your subconscious mind will automatically begin working on helping you achieve them. This is a powerful technique, and it works.

My goal is to apply to the _____PA program(s) and be accepted by _____. (Call each program that you will apply to and find out when candidates are notified about acceptance.)

In order to achieve this goal, I will have to overcome the following obstacles: (List all of the obstacles that you are likely to encounter: financial, relocation, convincing a spouse, etc.)

_____
_____
_____
_____

The following people and organizations will help me to achieve this goal: (List everyone who can help you along the way, i.e., other PAs, the AAPA, your state chapter of the AAPA, friends, relatives, and me.)

_____
_____
_____

To be a competitive candidate I will have to: (What will it take for you to stand out from the crowd? For example, will you have to take more science courses, gain more experience, work on getting a great letter of reference?)

_____
_____
_____

Beginning tonight, I will start putting into action the following plan: (Ask yourself what you can do right now to get started.)

_____
_____
_____

The benefits I will receive from achieving this goal of **getting into the PA school of my choice** include: (Ask yourself, "What's in it for me? Why do I want to pursue this goal in the first place?")

_____
_____
_____

The following is a list of synonyms that will help you add more life and power to your essays. I encourage you to purchase a book of synonyms and refer to it frequently.

articulate: crystal-clear, distinct, intelligible, eloquent, fluent, coherent

logic: sound judgment, presence of mind, foresight, wisdom

perceptive: sensitive, responsive, open, discriminating, insightful, quick, keen

enthusiasm: intensity, fervor, glow, fire, zeal, passion, spirit, vivacity, emotion

commitment: vow, assurance, obligation, guarantee, determination, promise

practical: wise, tough, judicious, prudent, shrewd, canny, sharp, astute, clever

crusader: fighter, visionary, advocate, champion, zealot, progressive

realistic: practical, pragmatic, common-sense, down-to-earth, sensible, rational

dependent: supported by, conditional, accessory to

tactful: diplomatic, prudent, discreet, sensitive, clever, skillful, polished

sincere: open, straight, earnest, fervent, dedicated, resolute, unpretentious

poised: composed, calm, cool, mannered, polished, suave, unflappable

integrity: honesty, veracity, candidness, honor

teamwork: collaboration, interaction, cooperation, synergy, harmony, concert

mature: refined, polished, self-sufficient, responsible, dependable, prudent

flexible: adaptable, conformable, adjustable, fluid, open-minded

Alabama Society of PAs
PO Box 550274
Birmingham, AL 35255
(205) 408-5757

Alaska Academy of PAs
PO Box 74187
Fairbanks, AK 99707
(800) 478-8684

Arizona State Association of PAs
PO Box 12307
Glendale, AZ 85318
(623) 582-1246

Arkansas Academy of PAs
950 North Washington Street
Alexandria, VA 22314
(877) 466-2272

California Academy of PAs
3100 West Warner Avenue #3
Santa Ana, CA 92704
(714) 427-03221

Colorado Academy of PAs
PO Box 4834
Englewood, CO 80155
(303) 770-6048

Connecticut Academy of PAs
PO Box 81362
Wellesley, MA 02481
(800) 493-9200

DC Academy of PAs
PO Box 50147
800 K Street NW
Washington, DC 20091

Delaware Academy of PAs
704 Dorcaster Drive
Wilmington, DE 19808
(302) 856-4360

Downeast Association of PAs
PO Box 2027
Augusta, ME 04338
(207) 629-9417

Florida Academy of PAs
PO Box 150127
Altamonte Springs, FL 32715
(407) 774-7880

Georgia Association of PAs
980 Canton Street
Building 1, Suite B
Roswell, GA 30075
(770) 640-1920

Guahan Association of PAs
PO Box 6578
Tamuning, GU 96931
(671) 646-5825

Hawaii Academy of PAs
PO Box 30355
Honolulu, HI 96820
(888) 942-2272

Idaho Academy of PAs
PO Box 2668
305 West Jefferson
Boise, ID 83701
(208) 344-7888

Illinois Academy of PAs
625 South 2nd Street
Springfield, IL 62704
(800) 975-9344

Indiana Academy of PAs
950 North Washington Street
Alexandria, VA 22314
(888) 441-0423

Iowa PA Society
200 10th Street, 5th Floor
Des Moines, IA 50309
(515) 243-2000

Kansas Academy of PAs
PO Box 597
Topeka, KS 66601
(785) 235-5065

Kentucky Academy of PAs
PO Box 23251
Lexington, KY 40523
(888) 884-5272

Louisiana Academy of PAs
8550 United Plaza Boulevard
Suite 1001
Baton Rouge, LA 70809
(225) 922-4630

Maryland Academy of PAs
PO Box 20277
Baltimore, MD 21284
(888) 357-3360

Massachusetts Assn of PAs
950 North Washington Street
Alexandria, VA 22314
(800) 441-2692

Michigan Academy of PAs
120 West Saginaw Street
East Lansing, MI 48823
(517) 336-1498

Minnesota Academy of PAs
4248 Park Glen Road
Minneapolis, MN 55416
(952) 928-7472

Mississippi Academy of PAs
PO Box 5128
Biloxi, MS 39534
(800) 844-4902

Missouri Academy of PAs
950 North Washington Street
Alexandria, VA 22314
(800) 844-4902

Montana Academy of PAs
1720 9th Avenue
Helena, MT 59601
(406) 499-7999

Naval Assn of PAs
950 North Washington Street
Alexandria, VA 22314
(888) 836-4169

Nebraska Academy of PAs
7906 Davenport St
Omaha, NE 68114
(402) 393-1415

Nevada Academy of PAs
PO Box 28877
Las Vegas, NV 89126
(702) 451-4578

New Hampshire Society of PAs
PO Box 325
Manchester, NH 03105
(603) 487-5248

New Jersey State Society of PAs
PO Box 1
Princeton, NJ 08543
(609) 275-4123

New Mexico Academy of PAs
160 Washington Street SE
Box 1
Albuquerque, NM 87108
(505) 342-8023

New York State Society of PAs
322 8th Avenue, Suite 1400
New York, NY 10001
(212) 206-8300

North Carolina Academy of PAs
3209 Guess Road
Suite 105
Durham, NC 27705
(919) 479-1995

North Dakota Academy of PAs
MSU Campus
Box 91
Minot, ND 58707
(701) 858-3848

Ohio Association of PAs
4683 Winterset Drive
Columbus, OH 43220
(800) 292-4997

Oklahoma Academy of PAs
PO Box 1132
Oklahoma City, OK 73101
(405) 271-2058

Oregon Society of PAs
PO Box 514
Oregon City, OR 97045
(503) 650-5864

PA Academy of Vermont
68 Overlook Drive
South Burlington, VT 05403
(802) 457-5000

Pennsylvania Society of PAs
PO Box 128
Greensburg, PA 15601
(724) 836-6411

**Public Health Service Academy
of PAs**
950 North Washington Street
Alexandria, VA 22314
(800) 441-3716

Rhode Island Academy of PAs
106 Francis Street
Providence, RI 02903
(401) 331-3207

Society of Air Force PAs
950 North Washington Street
Alexandria, VA 22314
(888)903-2272

Society of Army PAs
6762 Candlewood Drive
Fort Myers, FL 33919
(941) 482-2162

South Carolina Academy of PAs
PO Box 2054
Lexington, SC 29071
(803) 356-6809

South Dakota Academy of PAs
3708 Brooks Place
Suite 1
Sioux Falls, SD 57106
(605) 361-2281

Tennessee Academy of PAs
1483 North Mt. Juliet Rd
PMB #203
Mt. Juliet, TN 37122
(615) 443-3052

Texas Academy of PAs
401 West 15th Street
Austin, TX 78701
(800) 280-7655

Utah Academy of PAs
50 North Medical Drive
Bldg 528
Salt Lake City, UT 84132
(801) 581-7764

Veterans Affairs PA Assn
950 North Washington Street
Alexandria, VA 22314
(888) 905-2272

Virginia Academy of PAs
10301 Democracy Lane
Suite 203
Fairfax, VA 22030
(703) 691-8515

Washington State Academy of PAs
620B Industry Drive
Building 8
Tukwila, WA 98188
(206) 575-4633

West Virginia Assn of PAs
PO Box 3625
Charleston, WV 25336
(866) 889-8872

Wisconsin Academy of PAs
PO Box 1109
Madison, WI 53701
(800) 762-8965

Wyoming Assn of PAs
1260 West 5th Street, #62
Sheridan, WY 82801
(307) 674-6166

ALABAMA

University of Alabama at Birmingham
Surgical Physician Assistant Program
University of Alabama at Birmingham
RMSB 481, 1530 3rd Avenue South
Birmingham, AL 35294-1212
(205) 934-4407
http://www.uab.edu/surgicalpa

University of South Alabama
Department of Physician Assistant Studies
University of South Alabama
1504 Springhill Avenue, Suite 4410
Mobile, AL 36604-3273
(251) 434-3641
http://www.southalabama.edu/allhealth/pa.htm

ARIZONA

Arizona School of Health Sciences
Physician Assistant Program
Arizona School of Health Sciences
5850 East Still Circle
Mesa, AZ 85206
(480) 219-6040
http://www.ashs.edu

Midwestern University
Midwestern University
Physician Assistant Program
Office of Admissions
19555 North 59th Avenue
Glendale, AZ 85308
(623) 572-3311
http://www.midwestern.edu

CALIFORNIA

Charles R. Drew University of Medicine & Science
Physician Assistant Program
Charles R. Drew University of Medicine & Science
The College of Allied Health
1731 East 120th Street
Los Angeles, CA 90059
(323) 563-5879
http://www.cdrewu.edu

Keck School of Medicine of the University of Southern California
Physician Assistant Program
Keck School of Medicine of the University of Southern California
Department of Family Medicine
1000 South Fremont Avenue, Unit 7 Building A6-Room #6429
Alhambra, CA 91803
(626) 457-4240
http://www.usc.edu/medicine/pa

Loma Linda University
Physician Assistant Program
Loma Linda University
School of Allied Health Professions
Nichol Hall, Room 2033
Loma Linda, CA 92350
(909) 558-0495
http://www.llu.edu

Riverside Community College
Physician Assistant Program
Riverside County Regional Medical Center/ Riverside Community College
16130 Lasselle Street
Moreno Valley, CA 92551
(909) 485-6100, ext 4335
http://www.rccd.cc.ca.us

Samuel Merritt College
Physician Assistant Program
Samuel Merritt College
450 30th Street, Suite 4708
Oakland, CA 94609
(510) 869-6576
http://www.samuelmerritt.edu

Stanford University
Primary Care Associate Program
Stanford University School of Medicine
703 Welch Road, Suite F-1
Palo Alto, CA 94304-5750
(650) 723-8600
http://pcap.stanford.edu

Touro University Mare Island
Physician Assistant Program
College of Health Sciences
1310 Johnson Lane
Vallejo, CA 94592
(707) 638-5440
http://www.tumipap.us

University of California Davis
Physician Assistant
    Program/Family Nurse
Practitioner Program
University of California Davis
Department of Family and
    Community Medicine
2516 Stockton Boulevard, Suite
    254
Sacramento, CA 95817-2208
(916) 734-3551
http://fnppa.ucdavis.edu

**Western University of Health
    Sciences**
Primary Care Physician Assistant
    Program
Western University of Health
    Sciences
College Plaza
Pomona, CA 91766-1854
(909) 469-5378
http://www.western.edu

COLORADO

Red Rocks Community College
Physician Assistant Program
Red Rocks Community College
Campus Box 38
13300 West 6th Avenue
Lakewood, CO 80228-1255
(303) 914-6386
http://rrcc.edu/health

**University of Colorado Health
    Sciences Center**
Child Health Associate/Physician
    Assistant Program
University of Colorado Health
    Sciences Center
P.O. Box 6508, Mail Stop: F543
Aurora, CO 80045-0508
(303) 315-7963
http://www.uchsc.edu/sm/chapa

CONNECTICUT

Quinnipiac University
Physician Assistant Program
Quinnipiac University
Office of Graduate Admissions
    (AB-GRD)
275 Mount Carmel Avenue
Hamden, CT 06518
(800) 462-1944
http://www.quinnipiac.edu

Yale University
Physician Associate Program
Yale University School of
    Medicine
47 College Street, Suite 220
New Haven, CT 06510
(203) 785-4252
http://www.info.med.yale.edu/
    physassoc/

DISTRICT OF COLUMBIA

George Washington University
(Master of Public Health)
Physician Assistant Program
George Washington University
900 23rd Street, NW, Suite 6148
Washington, DC 20037
(202) 994-7644
http://www.gwu.edu/~gwu_pa

George Washington University
(Master of Science)
Physician Assistant Program
George Washington University
23rd Street, NW, Suite 6148
Washington, DC 20037
(202) 994-7644
http://www.gwu.edu/~gwu_pa

Howard University
Physician Assistant Program
Howard University
College of Pharmacy, Nursing, and
    Allied Health Sciences
6th and Bryant Streets, NW,
    Annex I
Washington, DC 20059
(202) 806-7536
http:www.howard.edu

FLORIDA

Barry University
Physician Assistant Program
Barry University School of
    Graduate Medical Sciences
11300 NE Second Avenue
Miami Shores, FL 33161
(305) 899-3964
http://www.barry.edu/gms/pa

**Miami-Dade Community
    College**
Physician Assistant Program
Miami-Dade Community
    College
Medical Center Campus
950 NW 20th Street
Miami, FL 33127-4693
(305) 237-4420
http://www.mdcc.edu/medical

Nova Southeastern University
Physician Assistant Program
Nova Southeastern University
3200 South University Drive
Ft. Lauderdale, FL 33328
(954) 262-1250
http://www.nova.edu/pa

University of Florida
Physician Assistant Program
University of Florida
PO Box 100176
Gainesville, FL 32610-0176
(352) 265-7955
http://www.med.ufl.edu/pap/apply

GEORGIA

Emory University
Physician Assistant Program
Emory University School of
    Medicine
1462 Clifton Road, Suite 280
Atlanta, GA 30322
(404) 727-7825
http://www.fpm.emory.edu/PA

Medical College of Georgia
Physician Assistant Program
Medical College of Georgia
Physician Assistant Department
AE 1032
Augusta, GA 30912
(706) 721-3246
http://www.mcg.edu/sah/phyasst/
    index.html

South University
Physician Assistant Program
South University
709 Mall Boulevard
Savannah, GA 31406
(912) 201-8070
http://www.southuniversity.edu

IDAHO

Idaho State University
Physician Assistant Program
Idaho State University
Campus Box 8253
Pocatello, ID 83209-8253
(208) 282-4705
http://www.isu.edu/PA prog

ILLINOIS

**Cook County Hospital/Malcolm
    X College**
Physician Assistant Program
Cook County Hospital/Malcolm X
    College
1900 West Buren #3241
Chicago, IL 60612
(312) 850-7255

**Finch University of Health
    Sciences/Chicago Medical
    School**
Physician Assistant Program
Finch University of Health Sciences/
    Chicago Medical School
3333 Green Bay Road
North Chicago, IL 60064-3095
(847) 578-3312
http://www.finchcms.edu

Midwestern University
(Master's Track)
Physician Assistant Program
Midwestern University
555 31st Street
Downers Grove, IL 60515
(800) 458-6253
http://www.midwestern.edu

Midwestern University
(Bachelor's Track)
Physician Assistant Program
Midwestern University
555 31st Street
Downers Grove, IL 60515
(800) 458-6253
http://www.midwestern.edu

Southern Illinois University
Physician Assistant Program
Southern Illinois University at
  Carbondale
Lindegren Hall 129, Mailcode
  6516
Carbondale, IL 62901-6516
(618) 453-5527
http://paserver3.som.siu.edu

INDIANA

**Butler University/Clarian
Health**
Physician Assistant Program
Butler University/Clarian Health
  College of Pharmacy and
  Health Sciences
4600 Sunset Avenue
Indianapolis, IN 46208
(317) 940-9969
http://butler.edu/cophs/

University of Saint Francis
Physician Assistant Program
University of Saint Francis
2701 Spring Street
Fort Wayne, IN 46808
(800) 729-4732
http://www.sf.edu/allied/pa.html

IOWA

**Des Moines University-
Osteopathic Medical Center**
Physician Assistant Program
Des Moines University-
  Osteopathic Medical Center
3200 Grand Avenue
Des Moines, IA 50312
(800) 240-2767
http://www.dmu.edu/

University of Iowa
Physician Assistant Program
The University of Iowa
5167 Westlawn
College of Medicine
Iowa City, IA 52242
(319) 335-8923
http://www.medicine.uiowa.edu/pa
  /pa.htm

KANSAS

Wichita State University
Physician Assistant Program
Wichita State University
College of Health Professions
Campus Box 43
Wichita, KS 67260-0043
(316) 978-3011
http://chp.wichita.edu/

KENTUCKY

University of Kentucky
Physician Assistant Program
University of Kentucky
121 Washington Avenue, RM
  118
Lexington, KY 40536-0003
(859) 323-1100
http://www.mc.uky.edu/pa/default.
  htm

LOUISIANA

**Louisiana State University
Health Sciences Center**
Physician Assistant Program
Louisiana State University Health
  Sciences Center School of
  Allied Health Professions
1501 Kings Highway, PO Box
  33932
Shreveport, LA 71130-3932
(318) 675-6937
kwilli6@lsuhsc.edu

MAINE

University of New England
Physician Assistant Program
University of New England
716 Stevens Avenue
Portland, ME 04103-7688
(207) 797-7261, ext 4529
http://www.une.edu/chp/pa

MARYLAND

Anne Arundel Community College

Physician Assistant Program
Anne Arundel Community
    College
School of Health Professions,
    Wellness and Physical
    Education
101 College Parkway
Arnold, MD 21012
(410) 777-7310
http://www.aacc.cc.md.us/ahd

Towson University CCBC Essex

Physician Assistant Program
Towson University CCBC Essex
7201 Rossville Boulevard
Baltimore, MD 21237
(410) 780-6159
http://www.ccbcmd.edu

University of Maryland Eastern Shore

Physician Assistant Department
University of Maryland Eastern
    Shore
Modular 934-5
Princess Anne, MD 21853
(410) 651-7584
http://www.umes.edu/pa/

MASSACHUSETTS

Massachusetts College of Pharmacy and Health Sciences

Physician Assistant Studies
    Program
Massachusetts College of
    Pharmacy and Health Sciences
179 Longwood Avenue, WB01
Boston, MA 02115
(617) 732-2140
http://www.mcp.edu

Northeastern University

Physician Assistant Program
Northeastern University
202 Robinson Hall
Boston, MA 02115
(617) 373-3195
http://www.bouve.neu.edu/
    department/pa/pap.html

Springfield College/Baystate Health System

Physician Assistant Program
Springfield College/Baystate
    Health System
263 Alden Street
Springfield, MA 01109
(800) 343-1257
http://www.spfldcol.edu

MICHIGAN

Central Michigan University

Physician Assistant Program
Central Michigan University
Foust Hall
Mt. Pleasant, MI 48859
(989) 774-2478
http://www.chp.cmich.edu

Grand Valley State University

Physician Assistant Studies
    Program
Grand Valley State University
Medical Education & Research
    Center
1000 Monroe Avenue NW
Grand Rapids, MI 49503
(616) 233-6500
http://www.gvsu.edu

University of Detroit Mercy

Physician Assistant Program
University of Detroit Mercy
8200 W. Outer Drive-Box 130
Detroit, MI 48219-0900
(313) 993-6177
http://ids.udmercy.edu/paprogram

Wayne State University

Department of Physician Assistant
    Studies
College of Pharmacy & Allied
    Health Professions
Wayne State University
Detroit, MI 48202
(313) 577-1368
http://www.pa.cphs.wayne.edu

Western Michigan University

Physician Assistant Program
Western Michigan University
1903 W Michigan Ave
Kalamazoo, MI 49008-5138
(616) 387-5314
http://www.wmich.edu/hhs/pa/

MINNESOTA

Augsburg College
Physician Assistant Program
Augsburg College
Campus Box 149
2211 Riverside Avenue
Minneapolis, MN 55454
(612) 330-1039
http://www.augsburg.edu/courses/
paprogram.htm

MISSOURI

Saint Louis University
Physician Assistant Program
Saint Louis University
School of Allied Health professions
3437 Caroline Street
St. Louis, MO 63104-1111
(314) 577-8521
http://www.slu.edu/colleges/AH

**Southwest Missouri State
University**
Department of Physician Assistant
Studies
Southwest Missouri State University
901 South National Avenue
Springfield, MO 65804
(417) 836-6406
http://www.smsu.edu/pas

MONTANA

Rocky Mountain College
Physician Assistant Program
Rocky Mountain College
1511 Poly Drive
Billings, MT 59102-1739
(406) 657-1190
http://pa.rocky.edu

NEBRASKA

Union College
Physician Assistant Program
Union College
3800 South 48th Street
Lincoln, NE 68506
(800) 228-4600
http://www.ucollege.edu/pa

**University of Nebraska Medical
Center**
Physician Assistant Program
University of Nebraska Medical
Center
984300 Nebraska Medical
Center
Omaha, NE 68198-4300
(402) 559-5266
http://www.unmc.edu/
alliedhealth/pa

NEW HAMPSHIRE

**Manchester Center for Health
Sciences of the MCPHS
Graduate PA Program**
Physician Assistant Program
Manchester Center for Health
Sciences of the MCPHS
Graduate PA Program
School of Health Sciences
1528 Elm Street
Manchester, NH 03101
(800) 225-5506, ext 4
http://www.mcp.edu

NEW JERSEY

Seton Hall University
Physician Assistant Program
Seton Hall University
400 South Orange Avenue
South Orange, NJ 07079
(973) 275-2370
http://gradmeded.shu.edu/school

**UMDNJ and Rutgers
University**
Physician Assistant Program
University of Medicine and
Dentistry of New Jersey and
Rutgers University
Robert Wood Johnson Medical
School
675 Hoes Lane
Piscataway, NJ 08854-5635
(732) 235-4445
http://www2.umdnj.edu/paweb

NEW MEXICO

The University of New Mexico
Physician Assistant Program
The University of New Mexico
    School of Medicine
Department of Family and
    Community Medicine
2400 Tucker NE
Albuquerque, NM 87131-5241
(505) 272-9678
http://hsc.unm.edu/pap/

University of St. Francis
Physician Assistant Program
University of St. Francis
4401 Silver Avenue SE, Suite B
Albuquerque, NM 87108
(888) 446-4657
http://www.stfrancis.edu/pa

NEW YORK

Albany-Hudson Valley
Physician Assistant Program
Albany-Hudson Valley
Albany Medical College
47 New Scotland Avenue, Mail
    Code 4
Albany, NY 12208
(518) 262-5251
http://www.hvcc.edu/paprogram

Bronx Lebanon Hospital Center
Physician Assistant Program
Bronx Lebanon Hospital Center
1650 Selwyn Avenue, Suite 11D
Bronx, NY 10457
(718) 960-1255

**Brooklyn Hospital Center/Long
    Island University**
Physician Assistant Program
Brooklyn Hospital Center/Long
    Island University
121 deKalb Avenue
Brooklyn, NY 11201
(718) 260-2780

D'Youville College
Physician Assistant Program
D'Youville College
320 Porter Avenue
Buffalo, NY 14201
(716) 881-7713
http://www.dyc.edu

Daemen College
BS/MS degree
Physician Assistant Program
Daemen College
4380 Main Street
Amherst, NY 14226-3592
(716) 839-8225
http://www.daemen.edu/
    departments/pa

Hofstra University
Physician Assistant Program
Hofstra University
113 Monroe Lecture Center
127 Hofstra University
Hempstead, NY 11549-1270
(516) 463-4074
http://www.hofstra.edu/pap

LeMoyne College
Physician Assistant Program
Department of Biology
LeMoyne College
1419 Salt Springs Road
Syracuse, NY 13214-4745
http://www.lemoyne.edu/pa/
    index.htm

**Mercy College Graduate Program
    in PA Studies**
Graduate Program in Physician
    Assistant Studies
Mercy College
555 Broadway
Dobbs Ferry, NY 10522
(914) 674-7635
http://grad.mercy.edu/
    physicianassistant

**New York Institute of
    Technology**
Physician Assistant Program
New York Institute of Technology
PO Box 8000
Old Westbury, NY 11568-8000
(516) 686-3881
http://www.nyit.edu

**Pace University-Lenox Hill
    Hospital**
Physician Assistant Program
Pace University-Lenox Hill
    Hospital
One Pace Plaza Room Y-31
New York, NY 10038
(212) 346-1503
http://www.pace.edu/dyson/
    paprogram

Rochester Institute of Technology
Physician Assistant Program
Rochester Institute of Technology
85 Lomb Memorial Drive
Rochester, NY 14623-5603
(716) 475-2978
http://www.rit.edu/~676www/main_pa.html

St. Vincent Catholic Medical Centers of New York, Brooklyn & Queens Region
Physician Assistant Program
St. Vincent Catholic Medical Centers of New York, Brooklyn & Queens Region
175-05 Horace Harding Expressway
Fresh Meadows, NY 11365
(718) 357-0500
http://www.svcmc.org

Saint Vincent Catholic Medical Centers of New York, Staten Island Region
Physician Assistant Program
St. Vincent Catholic Medical Centers of New York, Staten Island Region
75 Vanderbilt Avenue
Staten Island, NY 10304-3850
(718) 818-5570
http://www.svcmcny.org

Stony Brook University
Physician Assistant Program
Stony Brook University
School of Health Technology and Management
SHTM-HSC L2-424
Stony Brook, NY 11794-8202
(631) 444-3190, ext 6
http://www.hsc.sunysb.edu/shtm

SUNY Downstate Medical Center
Physician Assistant Program
State University of New York Downstate Medical Center
450 Clarkson Avenue Box 1222
Brooklyn, NY 11203
(718) 270-2324/5
http://www.downstate.edu

The Sophie Davis School of Biomedical Education CUNY Medical School at Harlem Hospital Center
Physician Assistant Program
The Sophie Davis School of Biomedical Education CUNY Medical School at Harlem Hospital Center
506 Lenox Avenue WP Room 619
New York, NY 10037
(212) 939-2525
http://www.ccny.cuny.edu

Touro College-Bay Shore
Physician Assistant Program
Touro College of Health Sciences
1700 Union Boulevard
Bay Shore, NY 11706
(631) 665-1600
http://www.touro.edu

Touro College-Manhattan Campus
Physician Assistant Program
Touro College-Manhattan Campus
School of Health Sciences
27-33 West 23rd Street
New York, NY 10010
(212) 463-0400, ext 792
http://www.touro.edu

Touro College-Winthrop University Hospital
Physician Assistant Program
Winthrop University Hospital
Extension Center Program 286 Old Country Road
Mineola, NY 11501
(631) 665-1600
http://www.touro.edu

Wagner College/Staten Island University Hospital
Physician Assistant Program
Wagner College/Staten Island University Hospital
74 Melville Street
Staten Island, NY 10309-4035
(718) 226-2928
http://www.siuh.edu/conindex4.html

Weill Cornell Medical College
Physician Assistant Program (a
surgical focus)
Weill Cornell Medical College
1300 York Avenue, Box 195
New York, NY 10021
(212) 746-5133/5134
http://www.med.cornell.edu/pa

NORTH CAROLINA

Duke University
Physician Assistant Program
Duke University Medical Center
DUMC 3848
Durham, NC 27710
(919) 681-3161
http://pa.mc.duke.edu/

East Carolina University
Physician Assistant Program
East Carolina University
School of Allied Health Sciences
West Research Campus, 1157
VOA Site "C" Road
Greenville, NC 27834
(252) 744-1100
http://www.ecu.edu/pa/

Methodist College
Physician Assistant Program
Methodist College
5107B College Center Drive
Fayetteville, NC 28311
(910) 630-7495
http://www.methodist.edu

**Wake Forest University School
of Medicine**
Physician Assistant Program
Wake Forest University School of
Medicine
Medical Center Boulevard
Winston-Salem, NC 27157-1006
(336) 716-4356
http://www.wfubmc.edu

NORTH DAKOTA

University of North Dakota
Physician Assistant Program
University of North Dakota
School of Medicine and Health
Sciences
Department of Community
Medicine
PO Box 9037
Grand Forks, ND 58202-9037
(701) 777-2344
http://www.med.und.nodak.edu/

OHIO

**Cuyahoga Community College
PA Program**
Physician Assistant Program
Cuyahoga Community College
11000 Pleasant Valley Road
Parma, OH 44130
(216) 987-5363
http://www.tri-c.edu/PA

**Cuyahoga Community College
Surgical PA Program**
Surgical Physician Assistant
Program
Cuyahoga Community College
11000 Pleasant Valley Road
Parma, OH 44130
(216) 987-5363
http://www.tri-c.edu/SPA

Kettering College of Medical Arts
(Post-baccalaureate Certificate)
Physician Assistant Program
Kettering College of Medical Arts
3737 Southern Boulevard
Kettering, OH 45429
(937) 296-7238
http://www.kcma.edu

Kettering College of Medical Arts
Physician Assistant Program
Kettering College of Medical
Arts
3737 Southern Boulevard
Kettering, OH 45429
(937) 296-7238
http://www.kcma.edu

Marietta College
Physician Assistant Program
Marietta College
215 Fifth Street
Marietta, OH 45750
(740) 376-4458
http://www.marietta.edu/
graduate/PA

Medical College of Ohio
Physician Assistant Program
School of Allied Health
Medical College of Ohio
3015 Arlington Avenue
Toledo, OH 43614-5803
(419) 383-5408
http://www.mco.edu/allh/pa

The University of Findlay
Physician Assistant Program
The University of Findlay
1000 North Main Street
Findlay, OH 45840-3695
(800) 472-9502
http://www.findlay.edu/academics/
    cos/phas/

OKLAHOMA

University of Oklahoma
Physician Associate Program
University of Oklahoma
Health Sciences Center
PO Box 26901
Oklahoma City, OK 73190
(405) 271-2058

OREGON

**Oregon Health & Science
    University**
Physician Assistant Program
Oregon Health & Science
    University
3181 SW Sam Jackson Park Road
    GH219
Portland, OR 97201-3098
(503) 494-1484
http://www.ohsu.edu/pa/

Pacific University
Physician Assistant Program
Pacific University
School of Physician Assistant
    Studies
2043 College Way
Forest Grove, OR 97116
(800) 933-9308
http://www.pa.pacificu.edu

PENNSYLVANIA

Arcadia University
Physician Assistant Program
Arcadia University
Brubaker Hall, Health Science
    Center
450 South Easton Road
Glenside, PA 19038
(215) 572-2082
http://www.arcadia.edu/default.asp

Chatham College
Physician Assistant Program
Chatham College
Woodland Road
Pittsburgh, PA 15232
(412) 365-1412
http://www.chatham.edu/
    academic/PA/pac1.html

DeSales University
Physician Assistant Program
DeSales University
2755 Station Avenue
Center Valley, PA 18034-9568
(610) 282-1100 ext 1415
http://www.desales.edu

Drexel University
Physician Assistant Program
Drexel University
College of Nursing and Health
    Professions
1505 Race Street, 8th Floor, MS
    504
Philadelphia, PA 19102-1192
(215) 762-7135
http://www.mcphu.edu

Duquesne University
Department of Physician
    Assistant
Duquesne University
John G. Rangos, Sr., School of
    Health Sciences
323 Health Sciences Building
Pittsburgh, PA 15282
(800) 456-0590
http://www.duq.edu/healthsciences

Gannon University
(24-Month Post-baccalaureate
    Master's Program)
Physician Assistant Program
109 University Square
Erie, PA 16541-0001
(814) 871-7474
http://www.gannon.edu

Gannon University
(60-Month Entry-level Master's
    Program)
Physician Assistant Program
109 University Square
Erie, PA 16541-0001
(814) 871-7240
http://www.gannon.edu

King's College
(Master's Degree)
Physician Assistant Program
King's College
133 North River Street
Wilkes-Barre, PA 18711
(570) 208-5853
http://www.kings.edu/paprog

King's College
(Certificate Program)
Physician Assistant Program
King's College
133 North River Street
Wilkes-Barre, PA 18711
(570) 208-5853
http://www.kings.edu/paprog

Lock Haven University
Physician Assistant Program
Lock Haven University of
    Pennsylvania
Lock Haven, PA 17745
(570) 893-2541
http://www.lhup.edu/academic/
    acad_affairs/academ_grad_
    phyas.html

Marywood University
Physician Assistant Program
2300 Adams Avenue
Scranton, PA 18509
(570) 348-6298
http://www.marywood.edu/ug_cat/
    departments/phys_asst.stm

**Pennsylvania College of
    Technology**
Physician Assistant Program
Pennsylvania College of
    Technology
DIF #123
One College Avenue
Williamsport, PA 17701-5799
(800) 367-9222
http://www.pct.edu/schools/hs/
    bpa

**Philadelphia College of
    Osteopathic Medicine**
Department of Physician Assistant
    Studies
Philadelphia College of
    Osteopathic Medicine
4170 City Avenue, Suite 005
Philadelphia, PA 19131
(215) 871-6772
http://www.pcom.edu

Philadelphia University
Physician Assistant Program
Philadelphia University
School House Lane and Henry
    Avenue
Philadelphia, PA 19144
(215) 951-2908
http://philau.edu/graduate/
    PhysicianAsst.htm

Saint Francis University
Bachelor's Program 60 Months
Physician Assistant Program
Department of Physician Assistant
    Sciences
Saint Francis University
PO Box 600
Loretto, PA 15940-0600
(814) 472-3020
http://www.francis.edu

Saint Francis University
Master's Program 24 Months
Physician Assistant Program
Department of Physician Assistant
    Sciences
Saint Francis University
PO Box 600
Loretto, PA 15940-0600
(814) 472-3020
http://www.francis.edu

Seton Hill University
Physician Assistant Program
Seton Hill University
Seton Hill Drive
Greensburg, PA 15601
(800) 826-6234
http://www.setonhill.edu/academics/
    index.cfm?ACID-114

SOUTH CAROLINA

**Medical University of South
    Carolina**
Physician Assistant Program
College of Health Professions
Medical University of South
    Carolina
PO Box 250856
Charleston, SC 29425
(843) 792-0376
http://www.musc.edu/pa_program/

SOUTH DAKOTA

University of South Dakota
Physician Assistant Studies Program
University of South Dakota
School of Medicine
414 East Clark Street
Vermillion, SD 57069-2390
(605) 677-5128
http://www.usd.edu/pa

TENNESSEE

Bethel College
Physician Assistant Program
Bethel College
PO Box 329
325 Cherry Avenue
McKenzie, TN 38201
(731) 352-4247
http://www.bethel-college.edu

Trevecca Nazarene University
Physician Assistant Program
Trevecca Nazarene University
333 Murfreesboro Road
Nashville, TN 37210-2877
(615) 248-1621
http://www.trevecca.edu

TEXAS

Academy of Health Sciences
Interservice Physician Assistant
    Program
Academy of Health Sciences
Attn: MCCS HMP
3151 Scott Road, Suite 1202
Fort Sam Houston, TX 78234-6138
(210) 221-8004

Baylor College of Medicine
Physician Assistant Program
Baylor College of Medicine
Room 633E
One Baylor Plaza
Houston, TX 77030
(713) 798-4619
http://www.bcm.tmc.edu/pap/

Texas Tech University
Physician Assistant Program
Texas Tech University Health
    Sciences Center
School of Allied Health,
    Department of Diagnostic &
    Primary Care
3600 North Garfield
Midland, TX 79705
(915) 620-9905
http://www.ttuhsc.edu/pages/alh

**The University of Texas Health
    Science Center at San Antonio**
Department of Physician Assistant
    Studies
The University of Texas Health
    Science Center at San Antonio
7703 Floyd Curl Drive, MC6249
San Antonio, TX 78229-3900
http://www.uthscsa.edu/sah/pastudies

**University of North Texas
    Health Science Center**
Physician Assistant Studies
University of North Texas
Health Science Center at Fort
    Worth
3500 Camp Bowie Boulevard
Fort Worth, TX 76107-2699
(817) 735-2301
http://www.hsc.unt.edu/education/

**University of Texas Medical
    Branch**
Physician Assistant Program
The University of Texas Medical
    Branch
School of Allied Health Sciences
301 University Boulevard
Galveston, TX 77555-1145
(409) 772-3046
http://www.sahs.utmb.edu/
    programs/pas

**University of Texas Pan
    American**
Physician Assistant Program
University of Texas Pan American
1201 W. University Drive
Edinburg, TX 78539
(956) 381-2292
http://www.panam.edu/dept/pasp

**University of Texas
Southwestern Medical Center**
Physician Assistant Program
University of Texas
Southwestern Medical Center at
Dallas
6011 Harry Hines Boulevard
Dallas, TX 75390-9090
(214) 648-1701
http://swnt240.swmed.edu/padept/

UTAH

University of Utah
Physician Assistant Program
University of Utah
375 Chipeta Way, Suite A
Salt Lake City, UT 84108
(801) 581-7766
http://www.utah.edu/upap

VIRGINIA

College of Health Sciences
Physician Assistant Program
College of Health Sciences
920 S. Jefferson Street
PO Box 13186
Roanoke, VA 24031-3186
(540) 985-4016
http://www.chs.edu

Eastern Virginia Medical School
Master of Physician Assistant
    Program
Eastern Virginia Medical School
701 W. Olney Rd., PO Box 1980
Norfolk, VA 23501-1980
(757) 446-7158
http://www.evms.edu/hlthprof/mpa
    .html

James Madison University
Physician Assistant Program
James Madison University
Department of Health Sciences
    MSC 4301
Harrisonburg, VA 22807
(540) 568-2395
http://www.jmu.edu/healthsci/
    paweb/paweb.htm

Shenandoah University
Division of Physician Assistant
    Studies
Shenandoah University
1406 University Drive
Winchester, VA 22601
(540) 542-6208
http://www.su.edu/pa

WASHINGTON

**University of Washington
    MEDEX**
MEDEX Northwest Physician
    Assistant Program
University of Washington
4245 Roosevelt Way NE
Seattle, WA 98105-6920
(206) 598-2600
http://www.washington.edu/
    medical/som/depts/medex/

WEST VIRGINIA

Alderson-Broaddus College
Physician Assistant Program
Alderson-Broaddus College
Box 2036, Alderson Broaddus
    College
Phillipi, WV 26416
(304) 457-6283
http://www.ab.edu

Mountain State University
The Physician Assistant Program
Mountain State University
PO Box 9003
609 South Kanawha Street
Beckley, WV 25802-9003
(800) 766-6067
http://www.mountainstate.edu

WISCONSIN

Marquette University
Department of Physician Assistant
    Studies
Marquette University
College of Health Sciences
1700 Building PO Box 1881
Milwaukee, WI 53201-1881
(414) 288-5688
http://www.marquette.edu

The University of Wisconsin-LaCrosse-Gundersen Lutheran Medical Foundation-Mayo School of Health Sciences
Physician Assistant Program
The University of Wisconsin-LaCrosse-Gundersen Lutheran Medical Foundation-Mayo School of Health Sciences
1725 State Street, 4031 Health Science Center
LaCrosse, WI 54601-3767
(608) 785-6620
http://www.uwlax.edu/pastudies/